DIABETES AS A WAY OF LIFE

BY T. S. DANOWSKI

Diabetes Mellitus with Emphasis on Children and Young Adults

The Body Fluids, Basic Physiology and Practical Therapeutics
(with J. R. Elkinton)

Clinical Endocrinology. I. Pineal, Hypothalamus, Pituitary and Gonads

Clinical Endocrinology. II. Thyroid

Clinical Endocrinology. III. Calcium, Phosphorus, Parathyroids, and Bone

Clinical Endocrinology. IV. Adrenal Cortex and Medulla

Outline of Endocrine Gland Syndromes

Sustained Weight Control: The Individual Approach

Diabetes As A Way of Life

Hypoglycemia Syndromes

Home Therapy of Diabetes Mellitus

DIABETES

AS A WAY OF LIFE

4th Revised Edition

T. S. Danowski, M.D.

Clinical Professor of Medicine, University of Pittsburgh
School of Medicine; Senior Staff Physician at
Presbyterian-University, Children's,
Shadyside and Magee-Women's
Hospitals of Pittsburgh; Consultant in
Metabolism, Veterans
Administration Hospital, Pittsburgh;
Chief of Medicine and Director of the
Institute of Graduate Medicine, Shadyside
Hospital, Pittsburgh, Pa.

Coward, McCann & Geoghegan, Inc.
New York

Patient care program described in the volume has been evolved with the aid of grants from U. S. Public Health Service, Dept. of Health, Education, and Welfare (Graduate Training Grants Program); Renziehausen Foundation of Pittsburgh; John A. Hartford Foundation, Inc.; American Heart Association, Inc., & State of Pennsylvania Department of Health, Division of Chronic Diseases, Section of Heart and Metabolic Diseases; Health Research and Services Foundation of the United Fund; The Pittsburgh Foundation (Charles A. Locke Educational and Charitable Trust); The Pennsylvania Lions Sight Conservation and Eye Research Foundation, Inc.; The Arthritis Foundation, Inc. (Western Pennsylvania Chapter); the American Cancer Society; and John and Rosalind Redfern.

Fourth Revised Edition, 1978

Library of Congress Cataloging in Publication Data

Danowski, T S
  Diabetes as a way of life.

  Includes index.
  1. Diabetes.   I. Title.   [DNLM: 1. Diabetes mellitus—Popular works. WK850.3 D188d]
  RC660.D28   1978   616.4'62   78-10197
  ISBN 0-698-10947-3

Second Impression

Printed in the United States of America

CONTENTS

FOREWORD

After ten years of guiding with his colleagues the care of as many as a thousand diabetic children and adults at the University of Pittsburgh Medical Center the author published a volume entitled *Diabetes Mellitus with Emphasis on Children and Young Adults*. This was written for physicians and specialists and is in most of its parts too detailed for even the paramedical professions such as nursing, dietetics, social service, etc., not to speak of patients. For our clinic and hospital diabetic care programs we had worked out a ten-page guide, in capsule form, for distribution to patients and their families. This outline, in keeping with the goals established in our clinics, provided the key information needed for satisfactory diabetic regulation. It made no attempt to present alternative points of view nor, restricted by its brevity, did it try to answer the many questions which naturally arise in the life or the mind of a diabetic.

The importance of filling the gap between two such information sources and meeting the needs of the millions of diabetics and their families becomes all the more important when it is realized that during more than 99 percent of his entire life span the diabetic and his family treat this disorder without a doctor, nurse, or dietician standing by. It is true, however, that handbooks for diabetics have been written in the past. Why, then, produce another?

The answer lies in the author's belief that diabetics and those around them desire ready access to all of the available facts about their condition. Diabetes is a way of life which contains all of the day-to-day problems and pleasures which make up the existence of any non-diabetic adult or child and a few of its own. These concern not only the types of food and the selection of insulins but the basic problems of growing up, employment, marriage, children and survival. In this volume the author has undertaken to discuss all aspects of diabetes, not "talking down" nor withholding facts. Alternative philosophies of treatment have been described and, although the program followed with our patients has been given in detail, no attempt has been made to prescribe for the individual patient. This approach is based on the premise that the diabetic who is secure in the knowledge that all facts as they are available have been made known to him is then in a position to cooperate intelligently and effectively with the physician responsible for his welfare.

T. S. Danowski

Pittsburgh, Pennsylvania

FOREWORD TO FOURTH EDITION

As the years pass more and more of the workers in the field of diabetes agree that prevention of high blood sugars will avoid or postpone some of the long-term changes in blood vessels and nerves which affect a minority of diabetics. Proof of this conviction awaits precise control of diabetes.

Hopes that transplants of pancreatic islets or a mechanical pancreas will provide such precise control remain to be realized but progress has been substantial.

In the meantime the author and others have been testing a program of self-measurement of blood glucose and four daily jet spray injections of insulin or variants thereof in attempts to control blood sugars of insulin-dependent diabetics completely. The results are encouraging but further tests are in order.

This volume is designed to guide you in your efforts to control your diabetes as completely as possible. Such control requires four elements, i.e. you, your family, your doctor, and knowledge.

T.S. Danowski, M.D.

Pittsburgh, Pennsylvania

DIABETES AS A WAY OF LIFE

1 : DIABETES AS A WAY OF LIFE

1. Are you alone?

Diabetes mellitus* can be defined as a condition in which the metabolism of foods in the body is altered. It is most readily identified by increased quantities of blood sugar or glucose in the blood and urine. However the metabolism of fats and of proteins is usually also changed, with decreased formation and increased loss of tissue stores of fat and proteins. Diabetes mellitus results from a shortage of insulin or a lack of the usual effects of insulin. In the United States

* Diabetes means "flowing through" and mellitus refers to honey, or in this case, sugar. It is to be differentiated from a totally different condition, diabetes insipidus, in which large amounts of tasteless or "insipid" urine are passed. For convenience sake, the single word "diabetes" is often used alone and in this case it always refers to diabetes mellitus.

today 5 per cent of the population has diagnosed or undiagnosed diabetes, or in total numbers approximately ten million Americans are diabetic. An even higher figure, 25 per cent, has been estimated for the inhabitants of North America based on the probability of an individual developing diabetes in the course of his or her entire lifetime.

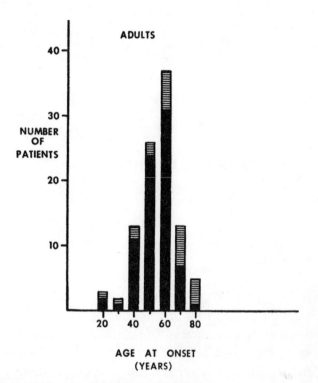

ADULT DIABETES: AGE AT ONSET OR DIAGNOSIS.

It is evident from the above figure that diabetes in adults appears or is first diagnosed most often during the 7th decade, i.e., in the 60's. This chart is based on a group of 100 of our patients in which there were more women than men. (Figure 1) Horizontal markings identify men.

Several reasons have been advanced for these differences. Heredity certainly plays a role, but composition of the diet, overeating and undereating are other important variables. However, there have been no definite conclusions reached as yet as to the exact prevalence of diabetes in various parts of the world and the factors which determine it. In American adults diabetes begins or is diagnosed most often in the seventh decade, i.e., the sixties, though of course no age group is exempt (figure 1).

The female sex is somewhat more susceptible than the male. This can only be partly explained by the longer life span of American women compared to men. The fact that females are more often overweight and that, under certain circumstances, female sex hormones influence the severity of diabetes, may also account for their greater susceptibility.

2. The emotional impact of newly discovered diabetes mellitus

The discovery of diabetes can be a painful emotional experience. Psychologically, practically none of us is ever really prepared for illness. This attitude of being "healthy minded" is normal, but it makes the shock of learning the opposite all the more difficult to accept. It is very important therefore to point out certain facts about diabetes which will eliminate needless fear and hasten the acceptance of diabetes as a way of life. Each diabetic who comes to us receives a brochure which we have prepared entitled "A Handbook on the Care and Treatment of Diabetes Mellitus in Children and in Adults." Various parts of it are reproduced on the pages which immediately follow and elsewhere in this volume:

This booklet explains what diabetes is and how it can be controlled. The name itself, *diabetes mellitus*, refers to the passage of excessive amounts of sweet urine. For hundreds of years this condition was but little understood and therefore feared. Now, however, a great deal more is known about it. While diabetes cannot be cured, its symptoms can be controlled and those with diabetes can look forward to long, useful, and healthy lives.

A. WHAT IS DIABETES?

To understand diabetes one must know how food is processed and used in the body. The ordinary complete diet contains carbohydrate, fat, and protein, in addition to minerals and vitamins. Carbohydrates, which include the starches and sugars, are the most readily available source of energy. Fat is a less rapidly absorbed but a more concentrated form of energy. Protein is made up of smaller units called amino acids and is essential in the structure and operation of all cells.

These three food elements, commonly called the chief foodstuffs, cannot be normally used, converted, or stored when diabetes develops. To understand this better it will be helpful to consider what happens to one of these foodstuffs, the carbohydrates, in the nondiabetic and the diabetic person. Almost all foods contain some form of carbohydrate. When the food is digested in the intestine the carbohydrate is converted to simple sugars and especially to glucose. This glucose is absorbed through the walls of the intestine and passes into the blood which carries it to the liver. Here and in other tissues it may be utilized directly, converted to fat or amino acids, or stored as another form of carbohydrate called glycogen. As the demands of the body require, the liver changes the glycogen back into glucose or produces sugar anew from protein amino acids and releases it into the blood for delivery throughout the body. The liver plays a key role therefore in the maintenance of blood-sugar levels. The cells of the body use this glucose as a furnace uses coal or other fuel. After it is absorbed into the cells its energy is released and the waste material, consisting of carbon dioxide and water, passes into the blood stream for disposal by the kidneys and lungs.

None of these processes can proceed at a normal rate without a hormone secreted by cells in the pancreas. This hormone, called insulin, aids in the storage of glycogen in the tissues and accelerates the use of sugar in the cells. There are other hormones and many other factors which influence the use of foodstuffs. For example, one factor important in the use of sugar by the body is exercise. The more work a person does the more sugar he will use, much like the furnace that requires more coal to heat a larger house.

When the body's supplies of insulin or the action of its insulin are insufficient, diabetes develops. The normal storage, use, and conversion of carbohydrate and other foodstuffs are upset. The liver releases its stored glycogen and produces increased amounts of glucose from the other foodstuffs. The cells of the muscles and other tissues which need sugar are unable to use it to a normal degree. As a result of this increased production and decreased utilization of glucose the amount of sugar in the blood rises to levels above normal. The cells are actually starving in the midst of plenty. They must call on another source of energy which does not require insulin. For this reason the fats of the body are converted into a form that can be used. In the process the body converts too much fat and the excess products accumulate in the blood as ketones which may also be referred to as "ketone bodies" or acetone.

When the level of blood sugar rises high enough sugar appears in the urine. The patient then passes large volumes of urine and begins to drink large amounts of water. If the insulin lack persists, ketone bodies appear in the urine and may result in acidosis. The patient may then begin to "overbreathe," i.e., to breathe deeply and rapidly, become very ill, and progress into a coma unless treated in the hospital.

B. HOW DIABETES BEGINS

Diabetes may appear gradually or suddenly at any age. Since there is a hereditary tendency, more than one member of a family can develop diabetes. The beginning may be marked by an increase in frequency and amount of urination and increased drinking and eating. It can follow "flu," measles, a cold or some other illness. There may be a loss of weight. In children body growth slows down, and the child may become irritable and begin to wet the bed again. In some cases there are repeated skin infections such as boils. In female patients itching often occurs in the genital area as a result of irritation by the sugar in the urine.

A simple test reveals the presence of sugar in the urine. A blood test taken while fasting, i.e., before breakfast or, better still, two hours after eating or after a test load of glucose (the latter is called the glucose-tolerance test) shows the amount of sugar in the blood to be higher than that normally found under such circumstances. Occasionally conditions other than diabetes cause glucose or other sugars to appear in the urine so that more complicated and lengthy studies are needed before a correct diagnosis is reached.

C. ATTITUDES

Before insulin was discovered, no child with diabetes ever lived to adult life and up to 60 per cent of the diabetics who developed diabetes as adults died in coma. Now insurance companies sell policies to patients! The well-cared-for patient can go through high school, college and university as successfully as the nondiabetic. He can choose any job, vocation or profession for which he is suited. If he, or she, finds the right one, marriage and parenthood can complete the picture of a healthy, successful life.

When the diagnosis of diabetes is made, the child and parent or the adult patient and his family must learn how to control it. This is done by giving a well-balanced diet containing the proper amount of carbohydrate, fat, and protein, by taking an oral drug or insulin, by testing of the urine for sugar and for acetone, and by encouraging normal physical activity. The overweight adult patient can often be treated by diet alone but some older adults and practically all young adults and children require insulin. The effectiveness of the treatment is determined by simple tests of the urine at home. Blood-sugar tests are not necessary as a routine and are reserved for special situations.

The child and adult patient should be directed toward a wholesome understanding of and adjustment to diabetes and encouraged to be self-reliant in living with it. For this purpose it is often helpful for the patient to be admitted to the hospital at the onset and at intervals thereafter. There the various necessary tests can be done as often as needed. A proper diet can be planned and the daily insulin need determined. At the same time the patient has the opportunity to learn as much about diabetes as he can understand from fellow patients and especially from nurses, doctors, and dietitians. During the hospital stay the patients and their families are also instructed in the management of diabetes. They are shown how to give insulin, test urine and prepare the diets.

Diabetes differs from many other illnesses in that control is a life-long daily procedure. It is best therefore that the patient learn to take care of himself as soon as possible. As the diabetic grows in knowledge, he learns to take over more and more of the daily details of diabetic life. Visits away from home, "eating out" in restaurants, vacations, and summer camp are as available to the well-instructed patient as they are to the nondiabetic, and are to be encouraged. With adequate training such patients, even the children, are usually able to assume complete responsibility in a surprisingly short time. The patients, the parents and the families then realize that those with diabetes can really live like other people provided they follow the simple rules of diabetic life.

3. The role of the doctor and of the patient and his family in the control of diabetes

The patient and his family require periodic reassurance that the diabetes is adequately regulated. The physician, provided with all the facts, can pass judgment on the point but this still leaves long intervals of time when the patient is on his own. It is then that a philosophy based on diabetes as a way of life is needed. Properly instructed, the patient knows just how far he can go on his own and when he must seek guidance. Here is our approach to the problem—but it is not the only one that is successful.

In our clinic and private patient practice we first try to convey all the understanding that we can to our diabetics. We do this in conferences and in quiz-and-answer sessions, in the guidebook or handbook already mentioned, and in urging membership in lay, i.e., "non-doctor," diabetes societies. Those present in or near your community may be found in the Appendix of this book. The patient is told all that is presently known about diabetes, and the most up-to-date methods of treatment and the still unsolved problems are described. Allowances are made for those who cannot for one reason or another assume any substantial measure of responsibility for their own welfare, but these patients are a minority. Again and again we have been impressed by the degree of understanding and co-operation shown by our charges, even the youngest of them.

What do we say to these patients? Throughout we tell them that diabetes is not to be considered a disease in the ordinary sense, since proper care will permit in most instances a long, useful, and normal life. Until recently the possibility that diabetes as we understand it today can be "cured" in the sense of certain other illnesses has seemed quite unlikely. However, the finding that pancreatic islet cells can be successfully transplanted experimentally after tissue culture and secrete insulin raises justifiable hopes that soon diabetes will be curable. In the meantime, diabetes need not prove a handicap to nor interfere with a full existence.

However, just as nothing in life is strictly black or white, it may not always be possible to attain ideal or perfect control in diabetes. In most cases it is a constant effort to reach this goal in the face of obstacles. These can be the result of chance (infections, accidents, or other illnesses), may be of our own doing (laxity in diet control, urine testing, unreasonable ways of life), or arise from natural phenomena (adolescence, menstruation, pregnancy, menopause). Hence, it is necessary for the patient to strive constantly for as complete control of diabetes as possible. It is the responsibility of the doctor to set as reasonable goals as possible for the individual patient. Not everyone can run a hundred yards in ten seconds or less, pitch a no-hit ball game nor be a tennis star, and, similarly, your doctor will not demand the impossible of you. He will expect, however, your very best effort and, far more important, ask you to demand the same of yourself. It is not enough to have sugar-free urine or a normal blood-sugar level at the time of the monthly or other visit to his office. What about the other 95 to 99 per cent of the time? And who is fooling whom if the patient "goes into training" just for the checkup?

The chapters which follow are designed to provide the patient and the family with facts, all of the facts, as they are available today. The reasons for and against each item of behavior are given as freely as they can be conveyed to you, because in the last analysis the most important factor, the indispensable ingredient, in regulation is the intelligent acceptance of diabetes as a way of life.

2 : THE SPECTRUM OF DIABETES

1. Diabetes in seven stages

The various types and forms of diabetes can be arranged into a spectrum. This spectrum begins before diabetes appears and includes temporary or stress-induced diabetes, milder permanent types, and the more severe categories. This spectrum consists of seven stages.

In Stage 1, also called pre-diabetes, diabetes pre-mellitus, or pro-diabetes, there is no increase, and there may never be, in blood sugar. Glucose and other tolerance tests are normal, and there is no sugar in the urine. In other words, none of the usual evidence of diabetes is present.

How then can we say that there is such a phase as pre-diabetes? We can make such a diagnosis with certainty, and only in retrospect, in persons who have already developed diabetes. Since they were not born with diabetes, it follows that they must have developed it after birth. Hence, pre-diabetes was present during some portion of the years between birth and the first appearance of diabetes. We know that such persons, before they develop diabetes, often have relatives with diabetes and are overweight. Also, there may be a history of large babies born into the family, or pregnancies may have been characterized by undue weight gain, swelling, and high blood pressure in the mother. Spontaneous abortions or miscarriages, death of infants before or shortly after birth, or babies with developmental defects can also indicate pre-diabetes.

In Stage II, or temporary stress-induced diabetes, the blood sugar becomes unduly high and sugar may appear in the urine as a result of stress and strain. The stress and strain can result from pregnancy; infection; injury; excess of hormones of the adrenal, thyroid, or pituitary glands; and drugs such as "water pills," taken to control swelling of the feet and other parts of the body, or birth control pills. The key to the identification of Stage II, or stress diabetes, is that it is temporary. When the stress ceases, the diabetes disappears. The person then moves back to Stage I, or pre-diabetes. However, stress-induced diabetes does not develop solely in pre-diabetic individuals. Thus, enough stress and strain such as severe infection and prolonged and marked hormone or drug excess can also produce temporary diabetes in a person without pre-diabetes.

However, if the discovery or the actual onset of diabetes coincides with stress and strain but the diabetes *persists* after the stress ceases, then this is classified as one of the further stages of diabetes, *viz.* Stages III through VII.

Stage III diabetes is the mildest and most common form of diabetes. It is so mild that in the fasting state the blood sugar is normal and the urine is sugar-free. The diagnosis of Stage

III diabetes is therefore based on the finding of an above-normal blood sugar after a meal or a sugar load. Sugar may or may not appear in the urine of such persons, depending on the level to which the blood sugar rises and the ability of the kidneys to filter and reabsorb sugar. Hence, absence of sugar from the urine does not exclude Stage III or, for that matter, any of the other stages of diabetes.

The mildness of Stage III diabetes indicates that the individual still has considerable ability to extract energy from and otherwise dispose of starches and sugar. Hence, the body has no trouble maintaining a normal blood sugar during the fasting or after-meal phase. The small amounts of sugar released from body stores or produced from protein during the fasting state or between meals are quickly consumed, and the blood sugar is kept within normal limits. However, when the load of sugar rises, as with food or during a sugar tolerance test, the mechanisms for the use of sugar are overwhelmed and the blood sugar increases above normal. Since the excess of blood sugar in Stage III is only present a few hours each day, it is often called chemical diabetes. However, it appears prudent to treat it as real diabetes because about one-half of the instances of persistent chemical diabetes are converted to obvious diabetes in the course of ten years. This can be prevented or postponed by anti-diabetic treatment.

In Stage IV diabetes the ability to handle even the small amounts of sugar produced or released during fasting or between meals is lost. Hence the blood-sugar level is above normal even when the person has not eaten for several hours or longer. The blood sugar increases even further after eating or after a sugar load.

The intensity of diabetes increases progressively in Stages V, VI, and VII. The increased intensity of the diabetes results from a progressive decrease in ability to use sugar as a fuel because insulin or its blood-sugar-lowering effect is largely or entirely lacking. Under these circumstances the body turns to fat for energy purposes because fat can be used as a fuel even when insulin or its action is deficient. It so happens, however, that when fat is summoned from body depots for fuel purposes, an excess amount is released. This excess, converted to ketone bodies, appears in the urine and may accumulate in the blood.

In Stage V diabetes, ketone bodies and acetone, which is derived from one of the ketones, are present in the urine but not in the blood plasma. This stage is usually called ketosis.

In Stage VI moderate amounts of ketone bodies have accumulated in the plasma and produced an increase in the acidity of the blood. This stage is termed keto-acidosis. The respirations usually become shallow and rapid, exceeding twenty-six per minute, as the body attempts to correct the acidity of the blood by reducing the plasma carbon dioxide.

In Stage VII diabetes, plasma ketone bodies are maximally increased and a more severe acidosis is present. Stupor or coma are frequent in Stage VII, and hence, this is often termed acidosis-coma. In this stage the respirations are of the air-hunger type, *i.e.*, deep and rapid.

In Stages V, VI, or VII diabetes the blood sugar levels are usually much higher than they are in Stages III and IV, and sugar is almost always present in large amounts in the urine.

Now it is important to emphasize that this spectrum is constructed from a total view of diabetes. The existence of such a spectrum does not mean that each person with diabetes passes through every stage of the spectrum. Indeed, only a very few, perhaps 1 out of 100, pass through to Stage V, VI, or VII and then with adequate therapy move back to Stage III or IV.

Most persons with diabetes do not pass beyond Stage III or IV and therefore have mild diabetes and huge margins of safety with respect to freedom from ketosis and coma.

2. Diabetes at various ages

Diabetes which appears in a child is usually strikingly different from that which develops later in life, *viz.* in the forties or fifties. Moreover, diabetes that arises in young adults in their twenties or thirties more often resembles the childhood form rather than the later onset or adult type. There are occasional exceptions to these rules. Thus, the childhood type may resemble that seen most often in older adults and vice versa. Usually it is possible to predict the characteristics of the diabetes in a particular person if the probable date of onset is known. These characteristics are of great importance to the doctor, the patient, and the family, for they provide the indications for a particular type of treatment and help the physician select the criteria for what is and what is not satisfactory control.

The approach of the adult types of diabetes, *i.e.*, Stage III and IV, is usually stealthy, while diabetes of the childhood type usually announces its arrival with a variety of complaints (see Chapter 14). Up to one-third of the children move into diabetic ketosis (Stage V), keto-acidosis (Stage VI), or acidosis-coma (Stage VII) ushered in by nausea, vomiting, abdominal pain, redness of the face, stupor, rapid or deep breathing, or loss of consciousness before the diagnosis is made.

Since the complaints which usher in diabetes are frequently preceded by a cold or other respiratory infection or a "virus upset" of the stomach and bowels, the presence of the diabetes may be masked. The parents may consider many of the complaints to be a part or an aftermath of the infection rather than an entirely new problem. This attitude can result in dangerous delays in diagnosing the diabetes. Medical attention may well be life-saving, since most of the deaths of children from diabetic coma occur in previously unrecognized and undiagnosed diabetes.

On the other hand, the stealthy approach of diabetes in the later years of life usually does not include any, or just a few, of the complaints which develop in children, and generally diabetic ketosis, acidosis, or coma does not develop. This reflects, of course, the mildness of the disease, even when untreated, on older adults. The diabetes of such adults falls into Stage III or IV. In the children, on the other hand, the diabetes is severe and can quickly, and often does, move to Stage V (acetone in the urine), or the life-threatening Stages VI (keto-acidosis) and VII (acidosis-coma).

The childhood and the late-onset types of diabetes differ also in the frequency of overweight present prior to or at the discovery of the diabetes. Judging from comparisons with healthy youngsters, most children who develop diabetes are of average weight and height or distribute themselves above and below these averages. Hardly any of them are fat. Indeed, when large enough groups of newly identified diabetic children are compared with their non-diabetic classmates, they tend to be a little below average in weight and perhaps in height. On the other hand, most persons with diabetes newly diagnosed in the later years of life (though because of its silence it may have been present but undetected for years before then) are clearly overweight. Indeed, if diabetes of late adult onset is not accompanied by overweight, it is apt to be more severe and resemble that which develops in children. Similarly, since diabetes which develops in young adults is generally not accompanied by excess body weight, it too tends to resemble the childhood type.

3. Body insulin in diabetes

For a long time, ever since the experiments which demonstrated that loss of the pancreas led to sugar in the urine, diabetes was attributed to a simple shortage of insulin. However, it was then realized that this explanation was inadequate when the diabetes required more insulin than the pancreas normally releases each day. To explain this paradox, inefficiency of insulin action was postulated in persons with high insulin requirements. Thus, it was suggested that anti-insulin factors in the body fluids or tissues reduced the usual blood-sugar-lowering action of insulin, or increased destruction of insulin interfered with the control of blood sugar, or overproduction of sugar was present. Some of these theories were tested and new ones were advanced once relatively simple methods for the measurement of insulin were developed. With such methods it is now possible to express in fairly precise mathematical terms the level of insulin-type molecules in the plasma of normal persons and in those with diabetes.

In healthy individuals the levels of circulating insulin are low during the fasting state. Food (sugars, starches, or proteins) or a glucose load quickly increases this level. As these food calories are consumed or stored, the insulin level quickly returns toward or to normal. In other words, there is a nicely timed decrease in insulin as the blood sugar falls. In this respect the level of blood sugar is quite analogous to the thermostat which determines the amounts of fuel which must be burned to maintain the temperature of a house within the comfort range. As this temperature is reached, the thermostat cuts off the flow of fuel and its conversion to heat. Just so, in health, the blood sugar level regulates the amount of insulin released by the pancreas to the circulation and in turn the rate at which blood sugar is consumed or stored.

Stimuli other than fasting and food also affect the supplies of insulin in health. Thus, physical activity reduces the need for insulin, while inactivity increases this need. Infections, emotional upsets, other hormones, the length of survival of insulin in the body, and undoubtedly other factors move the insulin need up or down.

In certain types of diabetes, such as that which develops in children, that which follows injury to the pancreas, or and then only rarely that which appears in the later years of life, there is an absolute shortage of insulin. In such persons the pancreas has lost its normal ability to manufacture and release an adequate supply of insulin in response to sugar or food. Thus, as mentioned earlier, most diabetic children have very little ability to make their own insulin when the diabetes first appears, and they almost always become incapable of secreting any insulin after a year or two of diabetes. Without treatment, these persons move into Stage V, VI, or VII diabetes. When insulin is not provided to such persons in adequate amounts, sugars taken by mouth or produced in the body cannot be used at a normal rate for energy or other purposes. The body then begins to rely on fat as a fuel because, in contrast with sugars and starches, its energy can be extracted even when insulin is totally absent.

Diabetes can be present, however, even when insulin supplies, judging from the levels in plasma, are just as high as they are in non-diabetic individuals. Also, food increases the insulin in these diabetic persons to levels as high as and often even higher than those attained in persons without diabetes.

Thus, in a minority of diabetic children and in virtually all late adult onset diabetes, insulin is still present but

       a)   It may not be released promptly, and/or

       b)   Insulin does not cut back the liver output of glucose which maintains our sugar levels between meals.

As a result the blood sugar becomes unduly high and when insulin is released it may result in below average, average, or above average insulin levels. The latter two categories follow upon the above cited delays or insulin inefficiency because of body fat, pregnancy, or certain hormones cancel out part of its capacity to enhance the use of sugar. In some the insulin receptors on the cell wall, to which insulin must bind before it can exert its effects, are decreased in number or defective.

This type of diabetes, in which insulin levels appear to be normal or even higher than normal and yet the blood-sugar levels are not controlled, is usually present, as already mentioned, in those who develop the disorder in their later years of life. Almost always such persons are overweight. These persons with diabetes of late onset almost always have mild diabetes in Stages III and IV. They can still extract enough energy from sugar to meet the needs of the body, and they do not therefore turn to fat as a fuel and hence do not form ketone bodies.

It may well be that the overweight in such individuals is perpetuated by the excess of insulin. The insulin does not possess its usual ability to control the blood sugar, but it still can and does promote the formation of new fat from sugar and from protein and interferes with the release of fat from body depots.

4. The search for diabetes

Many of the community surveys for diabetes and the routine blood tests during hospitalization are based on tests of the urine for sugar and measurement of the blood sugar while the person is in the fasting state or between meals. These tests will indeed identify persons with obvious diabetes in which the blood sugar is above normal even when food is not being absorbed (Stage IV diabetes), and at that time or after eating, sugar appears in the urine. Tests of this type however will fail, almost all of the time, to identify the milder form (Stage III) of diabetes.

Most of the time the diagnosis of diabetes in Stage III requires one or another of the sugar or food tolerance tests. These usually consist of measurements of the blood sugar before and at intervals of up to three or more hours after drinking or injecting a solution of glucose in water or after eating a meal or a specially prepared candy bar which contains sugar and starches in ordinary or in estimated amounts. Such a test identifies the person with hidden glucose or food intolerance. The presence of diabetes can be conclusively excluded only by means of an adequate glucose tolerance test. The tests based on a measured amount of glucose yield more precise results and are therefore used more often. However, in some persons useful information can be obtained with the food test.

The glucose tolerance tests are usually conducted in the morning with the zero-hour blood sample obtained after an overnight fast. In some institutions it is customary to instruct the person to be sure to eat ordinary daily amounts (at least 300 grams) of carbohydrate during the three days preceding the test. In the usual oral glucose tolerance test the person is given 3.33 ounces (100 grams) of glucose, or an amount adjusted for the body weight, *viz.* 1.75 grams per kilogram (2.2 pounds), as a solution in water. At times a smaller quantity is injected into a vein. These test solutions are taken or injected right after the zero-hour blood sample. Blood is then withdrawn from an arm vein (less often from finger capillaries) at the one-half, one and subsequent hours. This blood or the serum obtained from the blood is analyzed for "true" sugar and at times for insulin or other items. The interpretation of the test results is based on reference standards obtained from non-diabetic and otherwise healthy persons in the same age and body weight range who have undergone an identical test.

Thus, the World Health Organization states that diabetes is present if the third-hour blood sugar level following an oral glucose load is 130 mg% or higher. The United States Public Health Service states that diabetes is present if the zero- and third-hour blood glucose levels in the oral tolerance test are 110 mg% or higher, or if three of the following four abnormalities are present: the zero-hour blood glucose is 110 mg% or higher, the one-hour is 170 or higher, the two-hour is 120 or higher, and the three-hour is 110 mg% or higher (Table 1).

On the other hand, the British Diabetic Association advises that a diagnosis of diabetes can be made if, at any time prior to the second hour of a glucose tolerance test, the blood glucose level is 160 mg% or higher and the second-hour value is 110 mg% or higher. Fajans and Conn, applying their Michigan criteria, have suggested that blood glucose levels in a tolerance test that reach 160 mg% or higher at one hour and 120 mg% at two hours indicate diabetes mellitus.

The dilemma, i.e. which of the above five sets of criteria should be employed in interpreting the results of an oral glucose tolerance test, can be very simply resolved by applying our GTS principle. This is based on the sum of glucose levels in venous blood at 0, 1/2, 1 and 2 hours after ingestion of 1.75 grams of glucose per kilogram of body weight. When the GTS_{0-2hr} value is 500 or less, the probability that the test would be called diabetic by any of the five sets of criteria is essentially zero. When it is 801 or higher, all five sets of standards agree that the test is diabetic. Tests with GTS_{0-2hr} values between 501 and 800 are in the equivocal zone because the various criteria do not agree on calling the test normal or diabetic. When such equivocal results persist on repeat testing, they indicate chemical diabetes. If they are replaced by normal tests, they can retrospectively be classified as transient stress, illness, obesity, drug-induced, etc. glucose intolerance.

Hence, once the GTS_{0-2hr} value is known, the individual can be placed at a definite point on the diabetes spectrum of seven stages, i.e. prediabetes, stress glucose intolerance, chemical diabetes, maturity-onset type, or the juvenile and young-adult types with ketosis, ketoacidosis, and acidosis-coma.

3 : SIGNS AND SYMPTOMS OF UNSATISFACTORY AND SATISFACTORY CONTROL OF DIABETES

What criteria are used in planning a satisfactory program of diet, insulin or oral drugs in diabetes?

1. Blood and urine sugars and urine acetone as indices

Theoretically, the blood sugar should be the ideal index for judging the severity of diabetes and the adequacy of control. There are several reasons, however, why such measurements are not practical nor realistic for everyday use. There is the problem of obtaining a blood sample by tapping a vein or puncturing a finger not once but many times a day, the complexity of the chemical analysis which places the test outside the do-it-yourself category, the inconvenience and the prohibitive cost of laboratory studies—assuming there would be enough technicians available to meet the needs of several million patients day in and day out—and finally the tendency for emotional upsets and other factors to produce temporary or sharp changes in blood-sugar levels super-imposed on the diabetes itself. This does not mean, of course, that such studies are not valuable, even indispensable, in the diagnoses, in the treatment of acidosis or coma, during operations, and in a host of other circumstances.

Fortunately there is an alternative means of measuring the adequacy of control which avoids all of these problems and that is the analysis of urine for glucose. The reason for this is simple: under most circumstances when blood-sugar levels are too high (i.e., above the levels present without diabetes under the same circumstances) spillage of glucose into the urine results. With the lower values present without diabetes the urine remains sugar-free. This relationship can be considered similar to that of water spilling over a dam, though it is not, strictly speaking, identical. The scientists who work on the identification of the various mechanisms of the human body have even created a language of their own, using terms such as "filtration rate," "tubular reabsorption," etc., in describing this and other facets of kidney function. It is not our purpose to delve into this field but merely to point out that in using the analogy of a dam we are converting into everyday language an extremely complicated natural phe-nomenon. Though much is lost in such a simplification, enough remains to provide a basis for understanding how the urine can reflect levels of blood sugar and under what circumstances this index can fail.

In contrast to the complicated basic physiology the mechanisms of the test are remarkably simple. In the guide for diabetics which we give to our patients the following instructions are listed:

A. THE USE OF BENEDICT'S SOLUTION IN TESTING FOR SUGAR

Benedict's solution, containing blue copper sulphate, is used to test the urine for sugar. When sugar is present, it reduces the copper sulphate to metallic copper. This changes the color of the solution from blue to green, yellow, orange or red depending on the amount of sugar present.

a. Pour one full teaspoon (4 cc) of Benedict's solution into a test tube.
b. Drop 8 drops of urine directly into the solution; do not allow urine to run down side of the test tube.
c. Shake slightly to mix urine with solution.
d. Place test tube in boiling water for full 5 minutes.

Remove tube from boiling water, shake, and record the reduction at once, using the scale which can be obtained from your druggist; on this the percentage refers to grams of sugar per 100 cc (approximately 3.3 ounces) of urine:

clear blue or green	(no sugar)	− 0%	Insignificant losses of sugar
cloudy green	(trace)	− 1/10%	
olive green	(1+)	− 1/4%	
yellow green	(2+)	− 1%	Moderate losses of sugar
orange or brown	(3+)	− 1 1/2%	
orange red or brick red	(4+)	− 2% or more	Marked losses of sugar

The day-to-day Benedict's urine-test results in one of our adult patients satisfactorily controlled on diet alone are shown in figure 2.

Detailed directions for the use of other types of tests for urine sugar, including Clinitest®, Tes-Tape®, Chemstrip® and Clinistix®, have been included in the Appendix. It should be kept in mind that the color descriptions for reading the test results are only approximations and the actual reference scale supplied by the manufacturer should be used with each test. *They are not interchangeable.* It is to be noted that the 1+, 2+,

URINE TESTS RESULTS IN DIABETES CONTROLLED ON DIET ALONE.

(*Figure 2*)

3+, and 4+ rating with Benedict's Clinitest®, and Tes-Tape®, have their own percentage meaning. To avoid confusion it is best, therefore, to use the percentage rather than the plus-sign readings.

In terms of relative merit the Benedict's test is the cheapest but it is cumbersome. Clinitest® and Chemstrip® do not require boiling but care must be taken to keep the tablets or powder dry before use and to read the instructions for interpreting the test results correctly. The Tes-Tape® is extremely convenient and highly specific, reacting only with glucose and no other sugar, but cannot always identify values between ½ and

B. ACETEST® FOR URINE ACETONE TESTS

In many patients the physician will find it advisable to have the urine tested for acetone as well as for sugar. Acetone is a breakdown product of certain fatty acids (called "ketone bodies" because of their chemical structure) derived from fat. The origin and significance of urine acetone are mentioned in various chapters and discussed in greater detail in Chapter 9. At present it is sufficient to note that the presence of acetone in the urine indicates that the body is unable to derive sufficient energy from carbohydrate and is therefore calling upon its stores of fat for this purpose.

The Ames Company, Inc. of Elkhart, Indiana, supplies Acetest tablets. One drop of urine placed on a tablet produces a lavender-to-deep-purple color if acetone is present. A color comparison chart is provided and the results of the test are listed as:

1 + = trace
2 + = moderate
3 + = strongly positive or large

The Ames Company also provides a series of reagent strips to test for urine acetone, sugar and other materials. Thus, a Keto-Diastix® strip dipped into urine for 2 seconds yields an acetone reading in just 15 seconds and a glucose value in 30 seconds. Chemstrip® supplied by Bio-Dynamics of Indianapolis, Indiana, is available for the same purpose.

These tests indicate that ketone bodies are present in the blood and spilling into the urine. This condition is referred to as "ketosis" and may be a forerunner of diabetic acidosis and coma (see Chapters 2 and 9).

C. URINE TESTS WHICH DO NOT REFLECT BLOOD-SUGAR AND PLASMA-ACETONE LEVELS

Occasionally the urine tests may not serve as accurate indicators of blood-sugar or plasma-acetone levels either because the patient does not or cannot empty the bladder completely or because the level at which sugar spills into the urine has been raised by changes in the blood vessels of the kidneys. Such discrepancies present special problems which can only be resolved by close study of the individual patient.

2. Symptoms

The brief description in Chapter 1 of the chemical disturbances present in diabetes has to be extended to provide a basis for understanding the symptoms and signs which may appear in the inadequately treated patient. Diabetes results from a shortage of effective insulin which alters the metabolism of foodstuffs, i.e., of the carbohydrate, protein, and fat present in the food we eat or store in our tissues. The most readily recognized sign of this disturbance,

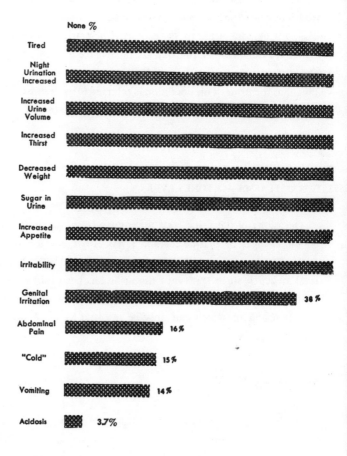

None %

Tired

Night
Urination
Increased

Increased
Urine
Volume

Increased
Thirst

Decreased
Weight

Sugar in
Urine

Increased
Appetite

Irritability

Genital
Irritation   38%

Abdominal
Pain   16%

"Cold"   15%

Vomiting   14%

Acidosis   3.7%

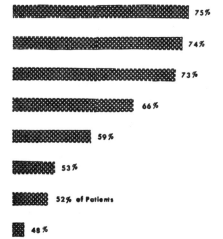

75%

74%

73%

66%

59%

53%

52% of Patients

48%

NOTE -21 patients without urinary symptoms at onset

SYMPTOMS AT ONSET OF DIABETES IN 100 ADULTS.

The fact that almost one-fourth of the patients had no urinary symptoms points to the need for regular check-ups of urine and blood-sugar levels if diabetes is to be detected early. (Figure 3) though by no means the only one, is the presence of increased levels of blood sugar before, during, and after meals. When these become high enough, sugar appears in the urine. At this point certain symptoms and signs may develop: losses of large amounts of sugar increase the volume of urine causing more frequent urination during the day and night, producing thirst, and leading to a greater intake of water. Because such losses of sugar decrease the calories available to the body the patients may lose weight even though the appetite and food intake are increased. They may complain of weakness, of feeling tired, or of being readily upset. There may be other disturbances present: the female patient may develop irritation of the external genitals, boils and skin infections may appear, and there can be changes in sexual function (irregularity or absence of menstruation and decreased sexual activity), and of sensations. Figure 3 summarizes the experiences of one hundred of our adults prior to the discovery of their diabetes. At that time, of course, the diabetes was unregulated or uncontrolled in each of these patients, but in many of the cases the diabetes was very mild. Among the hundred adults, one quarter could not recall any symptoms whatsoever which pointed to the presence of diabetes, and diagnosis was based on blood or urine tests. In the remainder the symptoms shown in figure 3 were present in varying degrees. Though not shown in the figure, overweight was frequent, occurring in more than 90% of the patients.

If diabetes remains unregulated it tends to become more severe. The body then relies more and more on fat for energy purposes since insulin is not necessary for its utilization. When the fat stored in tissues is mobilized, however, in excess of the capacity of the tissue to use it, ketone bodies, the products of fat metabolism, appear in the body fluids and urine, and acidosis and coma may result.

And what of the signs of well-controlled diabetes? In a sense there are none: the patient feels as well as he or she ever did prior to the onset of diabetes, lives a full and unrestricted life, and is, of course, free of the symptoms of unregulated diabetes.

In many clinics an all-out effort is made to keep the blood- and urine-sugar levels as close to normal as possible in the hope of avoiding some of the long-term complications of diabetes discussed in Chapter 12. In other clinics the emphasis is largely or entirely upon keeping the patient free of symptoms of diabetes. In still others a middle-of-the-road program is followed, i.e., an attempt is made to keep the patient as well regulated as possible without running the risk of insulin shocks and without imposing burdensome restrictions. Only the qualified doctor should decide which program is best for the patient under his care.

4 : TREATMENT OF DIABETES WITH FOOD

There are seven cardinal rules for the treatment of diabetes by diet. Thus, the diet must provide:

1. Enough sugars and starches to avoid starvation ketosis (100-150 grams as minimum);
2. Enough protein to allow growth and maintenance of tissues;
3. Only enough fat of the right type so that the total of calories from fat, carbohydrate, and protein will restore and maintain ideal body weight;
4. A proper distribution of protein, fat, and carbohydrate into three main meals and, if prescribed, two or more between-meal feedings;
5. Appropriate amounts of calcium, iron, vitamins, and other essential constituents;
6. An array of foods pleasing to the taste; and
7. A minimum of preparative, financial, and socially restrictive burdens.

It is of great importance to the patient to realize that many cases of adult diabetes can be treated merely by adjustments in the intake of ordinary foods. From the historical point of view it is now some fifty years since three Rockefeller Institute physicians, Drs. Allen, Stillman and Fitz, demonstrated that total starvation for seven to ten days with water allowed as desired improved the condition of seriously ill patients. In these studies they proved very dramatically that even the most severe diabetics possess a residual ability to convert foodstuffs stored in the body, even carbohydrate, into energy though they lack normal supplies of insulin. During this period of starvation these patients of course lost weight but the diabetes improved, as indicated by the lowering of the blood- and urine-sugar levels. After this initial period without food, they were given an adequate supply of meat and other protein, carbohydrate in the form of bulky vegetables within their ability to tolerate them without increases in sugar levels, and enough fat to provide energy. The patients did better on this program than on an unrestricted diet, though many still died in coma. At about this time however, Banting and Best announced the discovery of insulin and, except in some countries, starvation has been abandoned as a means of treating diabetes. In Germany and elsewhere on the Continent, however, some physicians still put their patients on one day of starvation out of seven. In the United States we continue to practice a modified form of starvation in overweight patients in that we cut down the total amount of food eaten. This not only reduces the load of food which the body must handle but at the same time decreases the need for insulin. These two factors are so effective that virtually 100 per cent of the definitely overweight adult patients whose body weight is reduced to normal can be treated completely by dietary restriction alone without insulin. The same desirable effect can be achieved in some adults with mild diabetes who are not overweight. Unfortunately it is not possible to treat most children by this method because they need insulin not only for activity but also for growth. In addition the residual supplies of insulin, or at least those amounts which reach the tissues in an effective form, are usually less in children than in adults. Hence insulin must be given to almost all children who have diabetes.

1. The prescription of diets for diabetics

In the handbook we give to our patients the general principles of diabetic diets are briefly covered in the following comments:

Growing children and adults need enough food of the right kind for health and growth and for replacement of tissues. In diets prescribed for patients the amount of carbohydrate, fat, and protein is specified so that it is neither too much nor too little. The total amount of the diet is based upon the patient's actual needs. The carbohydrates may be distributed in equal or unequal parts among the three meals depending on the insulin used, and some may be given as in-between-meal feedings. Younger children and some older diabetics need a midmorning snack. All patients should have midafternoon feedings and especially after exercise. Before-bed snacks are necessary in patients on long-acting insulin and make social eating at parties, dates, etc., possible.

With a proper diet a patient will not be tempted to eat extra food. If this does happen, the patient should not be scolded but the reason for the transgression determined. It may be that the diet is no longer adequate. As the child grows or the adult's caloric needs increase, the diet prescription is raised by the doctor. No patient should be unnecessarily hungry.

Meals should never be omitted. If the patient does not feel like eating solid food, substitutes should be given according to the exchange list. If rejection of food continues, or if vomiting occurs, phone the doctor at once.

In the early days following the availability of insulin a variety of diets were used insofar as carbohydrate, protein, and fat content was concerned. This necessitated calculations based on the average composition of foods and weighing of the individual servings. This is still the custom of most physicians and clinics, though the calculations have been greatly simplified by the exchange lists described in this chapter and by reliance on household measures (cup, tablespoon, etc.) rather than on scales. In prescribing a diet the physician or the dietitian under his guidance first determines the daily caloric needs of the patient, taking into account the physical activity and the need to lose or to gain weight. The ordinary young or middle-aged male whitecollar worker of ideal body weight takes about 18 calories per pound of body weight. Women usually take 10 to 20 per cent less. Thus a 150-pound man eats about 2,700 calories each day. In the diabetic diet these calories are prescribed with the following rules in mind: the carbohydrate is limited to 150 to 250 grams divided either equally or unequally among the three meals depending on the type of insulin used and dietary habits, about 1 gram of protein is given for each 2.2 pounds of body weight, and the remainder of the calories is obtained from fat. If the patient is a laborer with greater caloric needs or must regain flesh lost before treatment was started, a larger diet is given.

In overweight patients the calories may be reduced, though care is taken to provide at least 100 grams of carbohydrate and protein in the amount noted. In children the caloric and protein need is highest shortly after birth, averaging approximately three to four times the calories and protein prescribed for adults per pound of body weight. These requirements decrease with age, attaining the adult level in the teens.

Once the caloric need has been estimated and the carbohydrate, protein, and fat content calculated, the prescription is converted into weighed amounts or household measures of food by means of the exchange lists discussed below. However, if the patient complains of hunger or loses weight, the diet may be increased. Conversely, if a desired weight loss does not appear, the intake may be lowered.

2. The use of exchange lists in preparing diabetic diets

In 1950 the American Diabetes Association, the American Dietetics Association and the United States Public Health Service announced a simplified method for the preparation of diets. This was accomplished by listing in separate tables those foods which in weighed or household-measured quantities contained about the same quantities of carbohydrate, protein or fat. Since this permitted a ready substitution of one food for another, these were called exchange lists or exchanges. There are seven of these, one each for meat, bread, milk, fat, and fruit and two for vegetables.

In using these lists the physician, the dietitian or the patient converts the total number of calories into exchanges with the aid of tables which are readily calculated or are made available free of charge by manufacturers of insulin such as E.R. Squibb and Sons, PO Box 4000, Princeton, NJ. 08540, or Eli Lilly and Co., of Indianapolis, Indiana, 46206. Thus a 2000-2200 calorie diet consisting of 196 grams of carbohydrate, 120 grams of protein and 95 grams of fat has in it 12 meat, 3 fat, 9 bread, 2 milk, 1 Group B vegetable and 3 fruit exchanges. The Group A vegetables contain almost no carbohydrate and fat and very little protein, and therefore may be used freely in addition to the prescribed diet. The exchanges other than the Group A vegetables are then apportioned into meal servings (see sample menus). Similar tables can be obtained for diets ranging in calories from 1000 to 3900. Some sample tables are included in this chapter.

Often the carbohydrate is equally divided among the three meals except that some may be saved for between-meal and bedtime snacks. At times, because of the eating or work habits of the patient or the use of certain insulins, the prescription of carbohydrate may be unequal. Thus, less may be given at breakfast when long-acting insulins of the type described in Chapter 5 and in the Appendix are used.

With a little practice the patient or the family can readily abide by the diet prescribed by the physician.

3. Other views on diabetic diets

Recent studies have shown that the carbohydrate content of a diet can often be increased considerably without significant effect upon the urine or blood sugar or the dosage of anti-diabetic drugs. This is possible because these larger quantities of sugars and starches increase the insulin responses of the pancreas. This is not observed in persons, such as children, with marked restriction or absence of insulin responses.

It may be desirable in some patients with increases in serum cholesterol to reduce the total amount of fat in the diet and, insofar as possible, to replace saturated fat with unsaturated fat. The sugar content of such diets must be raised of course to maintain a constant intake of calories.

Some doctors have patients who are permitted almost unrestricted diets. This view that in certain patients liberalized programs work out satisfactorily arose naturally in the course of observing that patients who failed to follow the diet did not get into immediate trouble. Also, in studies in children made by Dr. W. O. Nelson and Dr. G. E. Guest of Cincinnati it was noted that, when allowed to eat at will from the family table, children ended up by taking about the same kinds and amounts of food present in the prescribed diabetic diets. Those diets are sometimes referred to as "free" or "normal," but not all physicians believe it wise to use them because control is not as perfect as possible. They feel that this may be a factor in the development of diseases of blood vessels in the kidneys, eyes, and other parts of the body which appear in diabetes of long standing. The decision as to the type of dietary program must therefore be in the hands of the patient's physician and should never be undertaken by the patient of his own free will or by default. It should be pointed out too that even on the so-called "free" program the diet must be as constant in calories and as well balanced with respect to carbohydrate, protein and fat as possible. The "free" diet is not a license to eat irregularly, to vary the amounts of food eaten day to day, nor to partake of items generally excluded from diabetic control programs such as candy, cake, soda pop, etc.

In general we urge our patients to use fresh fruits and vegetables. If these are not available, frozen fruits and vegetables prepared without the addition of sugar, or canned without syrup, may be employed. These dietetic canned fruits and vegetables are somewhat more expensive. The greater outlay is justifiable because the ordinary canned fruits, many of the frozen ones and certain of the canned and frozen vegetables contain large amounts of sugar and therefore would represent an unduly large proportion of the patient's allotment of carbohydrate. In an emergency, fruits canned with syrup may be washed with water to make up salads and deserts but this is not as satisfactory as the use of fresh or specially packed fruits.

The exchange tables in this chapter are based on material in *Meal Planning with Exchange Lists,* prepared by Committees of the American Diabetes Association, Incorporated, and the American Dietetic Association in cooperation with the Chronic Disease Program, Public Health Service, Department of Health Education and Welfare.

APPROXIMATE FOOD VALUES OF ITEMS IN EACH OF THE EXCHANGE LISTS

Group	Amount	Weight	Carbo-hydrate	Protein	Fat	Energy
		grams	grams	grams	grams	calories
Milk, whole ...	½ pt.	240	12	8	10	170
Vegetable, Group A ...	as desired	–	–	–	–	–
Vegetable, Group B ...	½ cup	100	7	2	–	36
Fruit	varies	+	10	–	–	40
Bread exchanges	varies	–	15	2	–	68
Meat exchanges	1 oz.	30	–	7	5	73
Fat exchanges	1 tsp.	5	–	–	5	45

MILK EXCHANGES

Per serving: carbohydrate, 12 grams; protein, 8 grams; fat, 10 grams

Type of Milk	Approximate Measure	Weight
	cup (8 oz.)	*grams*
Whole milk (plain or homogenized)	1	240
Skim milk *	1	240
Evaporated milk	½	120
Powdered whole milk	¼	35
Powdered skim milk (nonfat dried milk) *	¼	35
Buttermilk (from whole milk)	1	240
Buttermilk (from skim milk) *	1	240

*Since these forms of milk contain no fat, two fat exchanges may be added to the diet when they are used.

GROUP A VEGETABLES

Negligible carbohydrate, protein, and calories if one cup (200 grams) or less is used

Asparagus	Eggplant	Lettuce
Beans, string, young	Greens	Mushrooms
Broccoli	Beet greens	Okra
Brussels sprouts	Chard, Swiss	Pepper
Cauliflower	Collard	Radish
Cabbage	Dandelion	Sauerkraut
Celery	Kale	Squash, summer
Chicory	Mustard	Tomatoes
Cucumbers	Spinach	Watercress
	Turnip greens	

GROUP B VEGETABLES

Per serving: carbohydrate, approximately 7 grams but see below; protein 2 grams (1 serving = 100 grams)

Food	Carbohydrate Content
	grams/100 grams
Beets	8.0
Carrots	7.5
Onions	7.2
Peas, green (medium).....................	9.0
Pumpkin	5.1
Rutabaga	6.7
Squash, winter	4.9
Turnip	4.6

BREAD AND CEREAL EXCHANGES

Per serving: carbohydrate, 15 grams; protein, 2 grams

Food	Approximate Measure	Weight
		grams
Bread	1 slice	25
Biscuit, roll (2-in. diameter)	1	35
Muffin (2-in. diameter)	1	35
Cornbread (1½-in. cube)	1	35
Flour	2½ tbsp.	30
Cereal		
Cooked	½ cup	100
Dry (flake and puffed)	¾ cup	20
Rice and grits, cooked	½ cup	100
Spaghetti and noodles, cooked..........	½ cup	100
Crackers		
Graham (2½-in. square).............	2	20
Oysterettes	20 (½ cup)	20
Saltines (2-in. square)	5	20
Soda (2½-in. square)	3	20
Round, thin (1½-in. diameter)........	6–8	20
Vegetables		
Beans and peas, dried, cooked (Lima, navy, split pea, cowpeas)	1/3 cup	100
Beans, Lima, fresh	½ cup	100
Beans, baked, no pork.............	¼ cup	50
Corn, sweet	1/3 cup	80
Corn, popped	1 cup	20
Parsnips	2/3 cup	125
Potatoes, white—baked or boiled (2-in. diameter)	1	100
Potatoes, white-mashed	½ cup	100
Potatoes, sweet or yams	¼ cup	60
Spongecake, plain (1½-in. cube).........	1	25
Ice cream (omit 2 fat exchanges)	½ cup	70

FRUIT EXCHANGES *

Carbohydrate—10 grams per serving

Food	Approximate Measure
Apple (2-in. diameter)	1
Applesauce	½ cup
Apricots	
Fresh	2 medium
Dried	4 halves
Banana	½ small
Blackberries	1 cup
Raspberries	1 cup
Strawberries	1 cup
Cantaloupe (6-in. diameter)	¼
Cherries	10 large
Dates	2
Figs, fresh	2 large
Figs, dried	1 small
Grapefruit	½ small
Grapefruit juice	½ cup
Grapes	12
Grape juice	½ cup
Honeydew melon (7-in. diameter)	1/8
Mango	½ small
Orange	1 small
Orange juice	½ cup
Papaya	1/3 medium
Peach	1 medium
Pineapple	½ cup
Pineapple juice	1/3 cup
Plums	2 medium
Prunes, dried	2 medium
Raisins	2 tbsp.
Tangerine	1 large
Watermelon	1 cup

*Unsweetened canned fruits may be used in the same amount as listed for the fresh fruit.

MEAT EXCHANGES

Per serving: protein, 7 grams; fat, 5 grams

Food	Approximate Measure	Weight
		grams
Meat and poultry, medium fat (beef, lamb, pork, liver, chicken)	1 oz.	30
Cold cuts (4½-in. square, 1/8-in. thick). . . .	1 slice	45
Frankfurter (8 or 9 per lb.)	1	50
Fish		
Cod, mackerel	1 oz.	30
Salmon, tuna, crab	¼ cup	30
Oysters, shrimp, clams	5 small	45
Sardines	3 medium	30
Cheese		
Cheddar or American	1 oz.	30
Cottage	¼ cup	45
Egg	1	50
Peanut butter*	2 tbsp.	30

*Limit use or adjust carbohydrate (deduct 5 grams carbohydrate per serving when used in excess of one exchange).

FAT EXCHANGES

Fat—5 grams per serving

Food	Approximate Measure	Weight
		grams
Butter or margerine	1 tsp.	5
Bacon, crisp	1 slice	10
Cream		
Light, 20%	2 tbsp.	30
Heavy, 40%	1 tbsp.	15
Cream cheese	1 tbsp.	15
French dressing	1 tbsp.	15
Mayonnaise	1 tsp.	5
Oil or cooking fat	1 tsp.	5
Nuts	6 small	10
Olives	5 small	50
Avocado (1-in. diameter).............	1/3	25

The exchange tables in this chapter are based on material in *Meal Planning with Exchange Lists,* prepared by Committees of the American Diabetes Association, Incorporated, and the American Dietetic Association in cooperation with the Chronic Disease Program, Public Health Service, Department of Health Education and Welfare.

EMALE (SEDENTARY) AGE 16–30; OR (ACTIVE) 31–49 YEARS

000-2200 calories

OTAL DAY'S FOOD

IST	FOOD	AMT.	C.†	P.† (in grams)	F.†
	Milk	1 pint	24	16	20
A	Vegetables	as desired within limits			
B	Vegetables	1 serving	7	2	
I	Fruits	3 servings	30		
V	Bread exchanges	9 servings	135	18	
	Meat exchanges	12 servings		84	60
I	Fat exchanges	3 servings			15
ALORIES 2119		TOTALS ►	196	120	95

Note: If desired, patient may substitute skim milk for whole milk and
d fat exchanges (List VI).
† Carbohydrate, Protein, Fat.

2000-2200 Calorie Diet

| **MEAL PLAN** | | **SAMPLE MENU** |

BREAKFAST

	LIST
Fruit: 1 exchange (if tolerated)	III
Bread: 1 exchange	IV
Butter: 1 tsp. or 1 other fat exchange .	VI
Eggs: 2 or 2 other meat exchanges	V
Milk: 1 exchange	I
Coffe or tea, as desired	

BREAKFAST

Stewed prunes (2)
1 slice toast
1 tsp. butter
2 poached eggs
1 glass (8 oz.) milk

LUNCHEON

	LIST
Meat: 4 exchanges	V
Vegetables: as desired within limits ...	II A
Vegetable: 1 exchange	II B
Bread: 4 exchanges	IV
Butter: 1 tsp. or 1 other fat exchange .	VI
Fruit: 1 exchange	III
Coffee or tea, as desired	

LUNCHEON

½ cup (4 oz.) grapefruit
  juice
6 thin round crackers
Cold plate:
  1 hard-cooked egg
  1 slice bologna
  3 medium sardines
  1 slice salami
  Lettuce leaves
½ cup carrots
1 slice rye bread
1 tsp. butter
1/8 qt. vanilla ice cream
2 Graham crackers
Tea

DINNER

	LIST
Meat: 5 exchanges	V
Vegetables: as desired within limits ...	II A
Bread: 3 exchanges	IV
Butter: 1 tsp. or 1 other fat exchange .	VI
Fruit: 1 exchange................	III
Coffee or tea, as desired	

DINNER

Clear broth
5 ounces broiled steak
1 baked potato
  (2" diameter)
Lettuce and tomato salad
2 slices bread
1 tsp. butter
1 cup red raspberries
Coffee

BEDTIME

	LIST
Bread: 1 exchange	IV
Meat: 1 exchange.................	V
Milk: 1 exchange	I

BEDTIME

1 slice whole wheat bread
1 scant tbsp. peanut butter
1 glass (8 oz.) milk

FARMER OR LABORER

3700—3900 calories

TOTAL DAY'S FOOD

LIST	FOOD	AMT.	C.†	P.†	F.†
				(in grams)	
I	Milk	1 quart	48	32	40
II A	Vegetables	as desired within limits			
II B	Vegetables	1 serving	7	2	
III	Fruits	3 servings	30		
IV	Bread exchanges	11 servings	165	22	
V	Meat exchanges	13 servings		91	65
VI	Fat exchanges	28 servings			140
CALORIES 3793		TOTALS	250	147	245

Note: If desired, patient may substitute skim milk for whole milk and add fat exchanges (List VI).
† Carbohydrate, Protein, Fat.

3700—3900 Calorie Diet

MEAL PLAN		SAMPLE MENU
BREAKFAST	LIST	**BREAKFAST**
Fruit: 1 serving	III	½ cup orange juice
Bread: 2 exchanges	IV	2 slices toast
Table fat: 6 exchanges	VI	4 tsp. butter
Eggs: 2 or 2 other meat exchanges	V	2 fried eggs
Milk: 1 exchange	I	1 glass (8 oz.) milk
Coffee or tea, as desired		2 tbsp. heavy cream
		Coffee or tea

MEAL PLAN

LUNCHEON *(continued)*   LIST

Meat: 4 exchanges V
Vegetables: as desired within limits II A
Bread: 4 exchanges IV
Table fat: 4 exchanges VI
Fruit: 2 exchanges III
Milk: 2 exchanges I

DINNER

Meat: 6 exchanges V
Vegetables: as desired within limits II A
Vegetables: 1 serving . . . . II B
Bread: 4 exchanges IV
Table fat: 4 exchanges VI
Tea or coffee

BEDTIME

Meat: 1 exchange V
Bread: 1 exchange IV
Table fat: 2 exchanges VI
Milk: 1 exchange I

Note: 12 fat exchanges for use in the preparation of meals are to be added to the above (List VI).

SAMPLE MENU

LUNCHEON

4 broiled frankfurters
1 serving sliced tomatoes
2 small rolls or 2 slices bread
4 tsp. butter
1 cup baked beans
Stewed prunes (4 med.)
2 glasses (8 oz. each) or 1 pint milk

DINNER

6 ounces roast pork
½ cup spinach
½ cup carrots
1 cup mashed potatoes
1 cube cornbread
2 tsp. butter
1/8 quart vanilla ice cream
2 tbsp. heavy cream
Coffee or tea

BEDTIME

1 oz. American cheese
5 saltines
2 tsp. butter
1 glass (8 oz.) milk

LUNCH TO CARRY

Sandwiches:
    (1) 2 slices rye bread
        2 tsp. butter
        3 slices liver sausage
        Lettuce leaf
    (2) 2 slices white bread
        2 tbsp. (scant) peanut butter
        2 tsp. butter
        Lettuce leaf
1 small banana
1 pint milk

OVERWEIGHT DIABETIC ADULT

1000 Calorie Reducing Diet

TOTAL DAY'S FOOD

LIST	FOOD	AMT.	C.†	P.†	F.†
				(in grams)	
I	Milk (skim or buttermilk)	1 pint	24	16	
II A	Vegetables	as desired within limits			
II B	Vegetables	1 serving	7	2	
III	Fruits	3 servings	30		
IV	Bread exchanges	2 servings	30	4	
V	Meat exchanges	8 servings		56	40
CALORIES 1036		TOTALS	91	78	40

† Carbohydrate, Protein, Fat.

1000 Calorie Reducing Diet

MEAL PLAN		**SAMPLE MENU**

MEAL PLAN

BREAKFAST ... LIST

Tomato juice or stewed rhubarb,
  if desired: 1 serving .... I A
Bread: 1 exchange IV
Egg: 1 or 1 other meat exchange V
Skim milk: ½ cup (4 oz.) I
Coffee or tea, as desired

LUNCHEON

Meat: 3 exchanges V
Vegetables: as desired within limits .. II A
Bread: 1 exchange IV

SAMPLE MENU

BREAKFAST

1 serving stewed rhubarb
1 slice toast
1 poached egg
½ cup (4 oz.) skim milk
Coffee or tea, as desired

LUNCHEON

Cold plate:
  1 slice bologna
  1 slice salami

MEAL PLAN

	LIST
LUNCHEON *(CONTINUED)*	
Fruit: 1 exchange	III
Coffee or tea, as desired	

3 P.M.
Fruit: 1 exchange III

DINNER

Meat: 4 exchanges	V
Vegetables: as desired within limits. . .	IIA
Vegetables: 1 exchange	IIB
Fruit: 1 exchange	III
Skim milk: ½ cup (4 oz.)	I
Coffee or tea, as desired	

BEDTIME
Skim milk: 1 glass (8 oz.) I

SAMPLE MENU

LUNCHEON
  3 level tbsp. cottage
    cheese
  Lettuce and tomato
    wedges
1 slice whole wheat bread
1/8 (7" diameter) honey-
  dew melon
Coffee or tea, as desired

3 P.M.
1 small orange

DINNER
4 ounces roast beef
½ cup peas and carrots
Celery hearts and radishes
½ cup applesauce
½ cup (4 oz.) skim milk
Coffee or tea, as desired

BEDTIME
1 glass (8 oz.) skim milk

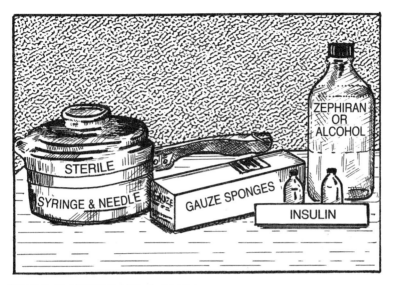

"SET-UP" OF STERILIZED NEEDLE, SYRINGE, STERILE GAUZE SPONGES AND
ZEPHIRAN OR ALCOHOL FOR INSULIN INJECTION.

(Figure 9)

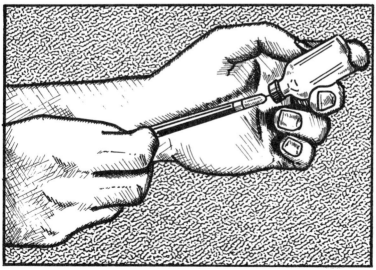

INJECTING AIR INTO THE INSULIN BOTTLE BEFORE WITHDRAWING
INSULIN.

(Figure 10)

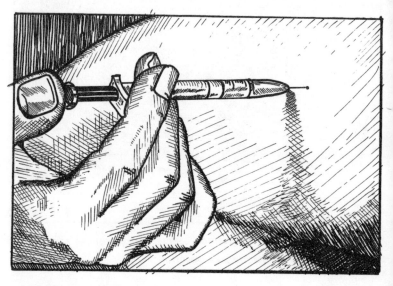

INJECTION OF INSULIN.

(Figure 11)

5 : INSULIN: A LIFE-SAVING CRUTCH

Prior to the discovery of insulin virtually all children with diabetes were doomed to an early death in diabetic coma and the same fate awaited 40 to 60 per cent of the adults.

1. The first isolation of insulin

In the summer of 1921 Banting, a Canadian physiologist later knighted Sir Frederick Banting, and Charles Best, a medical student, demonstrated that extracts from certain cells in the islets of the pancreas lowered the blood sugar of diabetic animals. In 1922 they first tested the material in diabetic patients. Within a matter of a few months a centuries-old problem was resolved. With insulin the blood sugar of unregulated diabetes decreased from its high levels and vanished from the urine. The chemical disturbances in body fluids could be made to disappear. New vistas of hope were opened. For the first time it was reasonable to believe that the dread of all physicians and the point of no return, acidosis and coma, might become just an episode. The extract soon granted life to untold thousands of hitherto doomed children and adults and substituted a reasonable intake of strength-giving foods for starvation. Truly a dramatic moment in the expansion of man's knowledge and one for which the world had been preparing for hundreds of years.

As in so much of human progress many had labored to prepare the way and to set the scene. The ancient Greeks and Romans recognized diabetes as an illness. Aretaeus of Cappadocia who lived in the first century. A. D. described diabetes as "a wonderful affection, not very frequent among men, being a melting down of the flesh and limbs into urine." The early microscopists undoubtedly saw the collections of cells in the pancreas which today are known as the Islets of Langerhans, named after the German pathologist and anatomist who described them in detail in his doctoral dissertation in 1869. Then two physicians, Oskar Minkowski and Joseph von Mering, working in Germany during the latter part of the nineteenth century, removed the pancreas of a dog and noted that large amounts of sugar appeared in the urine. For the first time diabetes had been produced experimentally. Yet despite this huge step forward more than three decades were to pass before an effective extract became available. These were years of anguish for scientific investigators who knew that the active principle was in some intimate way tied up with the pancreas. Yet all attempts to **lower the blood sugar by feeding the pancreas or products of** this gland proved unsuccessful. The same was largely though not entirely true of injection experiments. At times an effect was obtained, but it was inconstant and largely non-reproducible. We can now explain why these tantalizing glimpses of a principle that could lower the blood sugar were present so erratically: the external secretions of the pancreas, those which empty into the gastroinestinal tract, contain digestive enzymes which can destroy the product of the islet cells. In an intact animal or man the islet cells pour their secretions into the blood stream directly (hence the term internal secretion) thereby escaping the secretions produced by the rest of the gland. If the gland is ground up and extracted, the internal and external secretions become mixed and the latter destroy the former. The tantalizing glimpses of a decrease in blood sugar resulted from the action of internal secretion which had escaped destruction. In Banting and Best's experiments the tying off of the passages of the pancreas through which the external secretions flow was followed by destruction of the cells which produced these secretions. Then extraction of the organ yielded internal secretions of the islets which were not exposed to the digestive action of the remainder of the gland.

We now recognize this internal secretion as insulin, named after the Latin word for island. Its chemical structure is now entirely known. It consists of a series of building blocks called amino acids joined together into the complicated molecule which makes up a protein. Fundamentally therefore insulin in its make-up resembles the protein of the meat, fish, milk and eggs of our diet and it is easy to understand why the protein-digesting secretions of the pancreas and other parts of the intestinal tract destroy it when it is given by mouth or when it is mixed with the external secretions of the pancreas. There is, however, something special about the individual amino acids or their arrangement in the protein molecule of insulin that confers upon insulin the ability to lower sugar. This secret still remains locked in the mystery of the molecule but already some progress has been made in demonstrations that individual parts may possess some of the

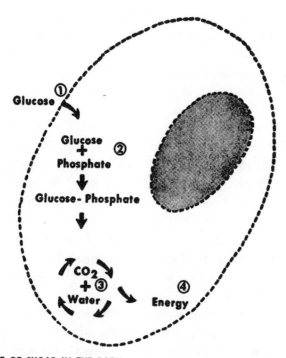

THE FATE OF SUGAR IN THE BODY.

The ovals represent a cell with its nucleus. The numbers 1 to 4 indicate sites where insulin may act, i.e., it may hasten the transfer of glucose into the cell, accelerate the union between glucose and phosphate, aid the breakdown of the glucose molecule to carbon dioxide and water or assist in the production of energy from the breakdown of glucose. (Figure 4)

activity of the whole molecule, and the entire insulin molecule has been synthesized in several laboratories.

2. How does insulin act?

Before beginning to point out how insulin lowers the blood glucose one must first explain the origin, changes and fate of sugar in the body. This is outlined in figure 4. In brief, glucose eaten as such or derived from foods or tissues enters into cells of the body and is either built up into a more complex molecule, glucose-6-phosphate, which can then be stored after further chemical rearrangements as glycogen in the liver, muscles and other tissues or which can be taken apart into simpler molecules that are ultimately broken down to yield carbon dioxide, water, and energy or converted to fat or protein. The numbers 1 through 4 in figure 4 mark points, established by laboratory studies, at which insulin may act to exert its effect. Number 1 in figure 4 indicates that insulin may merely serve as a key which opens the door. allowing glucose to enter the cell. This is an extremely attractive theory for which considerable experimental support has accumulated. It may be, however, that insulin also acts at site 2, expediting the union of glucose and phosphate, at point 3 helping the final breakdown of the sugar molecule into its component parts, or at 4 capturing and storing the released energy.

3. The seven types of insulin available.

Insulin comes in 10 cc* vials and each cc contains either 40 units (red lettering), 80 units (blue-green lettering), or 100 units (black lettering). However, to avoid confusion, the 40 and 80 unit vials are being phased out. In the case of crystalline insulin, 500 unit per cc vials are also available to meet special needs.

There are many different types of insulin in use throughout the world today. All of them are obtained from the

---

*CC refers to cubic centimeter (also known as milliliter or ml.), a unit employed in measuring volume and equal to 1/1000th of a liter. A liter is equal to about one quart. For purposes of comparison: 15 drops make 1 cc, a teaspoon of liquid contains 4 cc, and an ounce of fluid is equal to approximately 30 cc.

TABLE I

Appearance and properties of various insulins

	Regular or crystalline	Globin	Protamine zinc	NPH	Lente*
Bottle	Round	Round	Round	Square	Six-sided
Appearance	Clear	Clear	Cloudy	Cloudy	Cloudy
Intensity of action	High	Intermediate	Low	Intermediate	Intermediate
Duration of action (hours)	8–10	14–18	24	14–18	14–18
	(short)	(intermediate)	(long)	(intermediate)	(intermediate)

*Semi-Lente and Ultra-Lente insulins which act more rapidly and less rapidly, respectively, than Lente insulin are also available.

pancreas of animals and all consist of a solution or suspension of insulin protein in water. Some are clear in appearance and others cloudy. Alterations in the molecule, produced by adding other proteins and metallic ions or various salts which change the physical properties and the rate of absorption of insulin, determine the onset and duration of action of the various types. In table I the appearance and properties of the insulins in common use have been summarized. A detailed discussion of the individual insulins has been included in the Appendix so that the reader interested in a particular type may have ready access to the available information.

It is useful however to keep in mind the fact that insulins may be grouped into three general classes:

1. Rapid Onset: Short Duration of Action Insulins
2. Slow Onset: Long Duration of Action Insulins
3. Insulin with Onset and Duration of Action Intermediate to 1 and 2.

This classification is based upon the rapidity with which the effect on blood sugar begins, the degree of this change, and the duration of this insulin action. Figures 5, 6, 7, and 8 are helpful in visualizing these properties. The dotted line identifies the range of blood sugar in healthy nondiabetics in relation to the meals. The shaded lines illustrate the course of the blood sugar in patients untreated and treated with various types of insulin. The arrow, when present, points to the time of insulin injection, usually 20 minutes to a half-hour before breakfast in the case of the rapid-onset short-acting insulins when used alone, and 30 to 45 minutes before breakfast in the others.

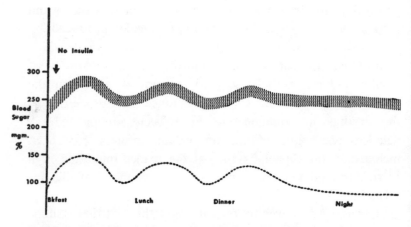

BLOOD SUGAR CURVES IN NONDIABETIC AND DIABETIC ADULT.

(*Figure 5*)

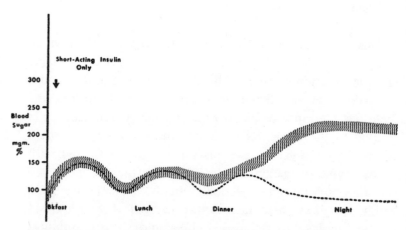

THE BLOOD SUGAR LOWERING EFFECT OF SHORT-ACTING INSULIN.

(*Figure 6*)

From figure 5 it is seen that in diabetics and nondiabetics the blood sugar rises after each meal as food is absorbed. The rise is greater and lasts longer in diabetes and sugar appears in the urine. Such a patient is losing calories and may have symptoms of uncontrolled diabetes, such as increased thirst and urination.

Figure 6 illustrates that a rapid-onset, short-acting insulin such as crystalline or regular starts working in about 20 to 30 minutes and has a peak action of about 4 hours and is used up at the end of 8 hours. Hence the blood sugar can be satisfactorily controlled during the early part of the day but rises to high levels after supper. This could be prevented by a second dose of insulin before supper.

From figure 7 it is evident that long-acting insulins used alone do lower the before-meal and after-meal blood sugar somewhat but the slow onset of action and the occurrence of a peak of activity at 12 to 18 hours does not fully control the after-meal spillage. This may not be a major problem in some patients.

Figure 8 shows that a combination of rapid-onset, short-acting insulin and slow-onset, long-acting insulin permits complete control 24 hours a day. This can be achieved with mixtures of crystalline and protamine zinc insulins, crystalline and NPH, crystalline and globin, with lente alone or in combination with crystalline, or with semi-lente or ultra-lente. (See table 5—1 and Appendix for further details about these insulins.)

4. Which insulin is best?

The selection of any one insulin as most suitable for all or even a majority of patients would be like saying that 8½D is

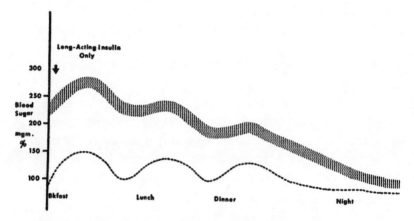

THE BLOOD SUGAR LOWERING EFFECT OF LONG-ACTING INSULIN.

(*Figure 7*)

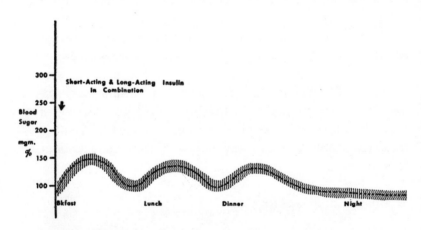

NORMAL BLOOD SUGAR CURVES WITH INJECTION OF SHORT- AND LONG-ACTING INSULINS.

(*Figure 8*)

the best shoe size for all or most people. The particular type used and the dosage and schedule employed should be just as individualized as the fitting of a shoe. Though insulin itself, no matter the form in which it is prepared, is a marvelous life-saving drug, the custom tailoring of its properties which the chemist has achieved necessitates and deserves custom fitting. Here a neutral expert, the doctor, rather than the patient, plays the key role.

5. The first dose of insulin

Like the first plunge into a cold pool on a rainy day, the first dose of insulin involves some hesitation on both the part of the patient and his doctor. The patient hopes that if he must have diabetes, at least may it not be necessary to take insulin. The doctor's uncertainty is not based on whether or not but on what kind and how much. The physician's knowledge of danger signs, such as symptoms uncontrollable by diet and signs of impending or actual ketosis or acidosis-coma, clearly provide the answer about the need for insulin. His own experience and that reported in the medical literature point to which insulin or combination of insulins is most likely to meet the needs of a particular patient of a certain age, body weight, energy requirement, etc.

However, only trial and error, and trial and error alone, will determine the exact amount of insulin which must be given to a particular patient. Neither the knowledge of the needs of a thousand other patients, the level of repeated blood-sugar examinations, nor the results of many urine analyses can be converted by any known formula into the number of units of insulin that the patient will need. We have to dispense with a common fallacy that, with a green

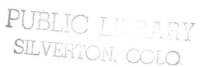

Benedict's urine test, take 10 units of insulin; with an orange-red test take 20, etc. The doctor tackles the problem by administering an amount of insulin which he considers to be safe and then determines its effect by the results of urine examinations and, at times, the findings on blood-sugar analyses. If the patient is in the hospital, all of the urine passed during a 24-hour period is saved and apportioned into collections which in the case of our patients extend between 8:00–11:00 A.M., 11:00 A.M.–4:00 P.M., 4:00–10:00 P.M., 10:00 P.M.–6:00 A.M. and 6:00–8:00 A.M. when meals are served at 8:30 A.M., 12 noon, and 5:00 P.M. If the urine tests show very little sugar and blood-sugar levels are not high, treatment may be confined to diet. If the patient is older and has a relatively mild diabetes a single dose of long-acting or intermediate insulins such as protamine zinc, globin, NPH, or lente insulin is tried. If the after-meal spill of sugar in the urine or the rise in blood sugar continues to be high, short-acting insulin is combined with the longer-acting insulins. In some clinics the two insulins may be given in separate syringes into separate sites but usually they are combined, sometimes even premixed in a bottle, and given at one time. The instructions we have prepared for our patients summarize how the doctor or his nurse and the trained patient go about administering insulin and adjusting the dosage in accord with the results of urine tests.

Keeping a record of the daily urine tests helps in determining whether or not the insulin dose should be changed. The urine is tested for sugar before breakfast, before lunch, before supper, and before going to bed. However, the urine that is first passed upon arising has collected in the bladder during the night. A test of this urine will therefore be influenced by any sugar passed through the night. For this reason it is best to test a second specimen as well. The patient should empty the bladder at once upon rising. After getting washed and dressed, a second specimen should be obtained and used for the test before breakfast. This urine will contain any sugar passed in the morning and the two tests will provide a complete guide to the action of the longer-acting insulin injected the day before. The test before supper serves as a dependable guide for regulating the dose of the crystalline or regular, i.e., rapid-acting, insulin.

If urine sugar is 4+ for two or more days in—
   a. before-supper specimen: raise regular insulin.
   b. second specimen before breakfast: raise the longer acting insulin.

If urine sugar is negative for two or more days in—
   a. before-supper specimen: lower regular insulin.
   b. second specimen before breakfast: lower the longer-acting insulin.

It is usually wise to raise or to lower insulin not more than two or three units at a time, not oftener than every two or three days. However, if the total insulin dosage is large, i.e., in excess of 50 units per day, the change may be as high as 5 or 10 units. Also, if symptoms of uncontrolled diabetes appear or acetone is present in the urine, the dosage may have to be changed to a greater extent and more rapidly. This should be done under the guidance of a physician. This is especially true when illness occurs.

In addition to recording the results of urine tests, always list the dose of insulin and any incidents such as insulin reactions, infections, menstrual periods, trips away from home, emotional upsets, etc., on the sheet provided for that purpose. The child with diabetes should, of course, do these tests and record the results as soon as he is able.

A record prepared by one of our patients in accordance with these instructions is shown in this chapter as figure 12.

The Injection of Insulin (Figures 9, 10, 11)

Insulin may be injected beneath the skin of the anterior-lateral thighs, upper arms, or the buttocks, using a different spot each day. By using six different spots in each area, no spot is used oftener than once in 36 days. Changing the site of injection minimizes swelling and may help prevent the opposite, *i.e.,* atrophy or loss of fat from under the skin.* Injection of the insulin deep into a muscle rather than under the skin will also eliminate the swelling or the loss of tissue.

Equipment

    a. Bottle of insulin as prescribed by physician.
    b. Aqueous zephiran, 1:1000.
    c. Cotton.
    d. Insulin syringe.
    e. Hypodermic needles, two, 26 gauge, ½ inch long.

How to Sterilize Needles and Syringes:

    a. Cleanse syringe and needles thoroughly with cold water. To clean needles, attach to syringe and force water through them.
    b. Separate plunger (inner part of the syringe) from the outer barrel.
    c. Put barrel of syringe and plunger in water and boil ten minutes

---

* It may be desirable not to rotate sites of insulin injection if localized loss of fatty tissue is occurring. This would then minimize the reaction to one area.

in a clean covered saucepan.

d. Drain water.

e. Replace lid until ready to use.

(None of these steps is necessary if a sterile disposable syringe and needle are used for each injection.)

How to Withdraw Insulin:

a. Use the U-40 insulin syringe for U 40 insulin; use the U-80 insulin syringe for U 80 insulin, etc.

b. Rub cap of insulin bottle with cotton wet with zephiran.

*c. Remove barrel of syringe from container in which it was boiled. Grasp only in the center. *Do not touch ends.*

*d. Remove plunger from container, grasping at top end; insert plunger into barrel of the syringe.

e. Remove needles from container; attach needle firmly to syringe, being careful to keep point and shaft completely sterile.

f. Inject as much air as the amount of long-acting insulin needed into the vial of the long-acting insulin and withdraw needle without insulin.

g. Inject as much air as the amount of regular insulin needed into the vial of regular insulin.

h. Turn the vial of regular insulin upside down and draw the proper amount of insulin into the syringe.

i. Turn the long-acting insulin vial upside down and draw out the insulin the proper amount. The total of the two types of insulin will be your final dosage. For example, 30 U regular insulin plus 15 U long-acting insulin will end up at the 45 U mark.

j. Inject the insulin under the skin or into muscle.

* Not necessary if a sterile disposable syringe is used.

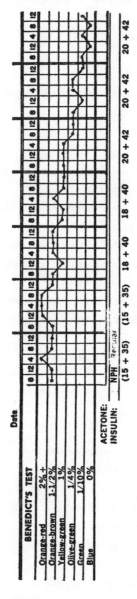

Date

BENEDICT'S TEST																						
Orange-red	2%+																					
Orange-brown	1-1/2%																					
Yellow-green	1%																					
Olive-green	1/4%																					
Green	1/10%																					
Blue	0%																					

ACETONE:
INSULIN: NPH Regular

(15 + 35) (15 + 35) 18 + 40 18 + 40 20 + 42 20 + 42 20 + 42

ADJUSTMENTS IN INSULIN DOSAGE IN ACCORD WITH RESULTS OF URINE SUGAR TESTS.

It is to be noted that excesses of urine sugar present in before-breakfast specimen require an increase in the intermediate insulin (NPH in this instance) and that a heavy spill of sugar before supper is controlled by raising the dosage of short-acting insulin. If tests remain negative, it is wise to reduce both insulins slightly to avoid danger of shocking. (Figure 12).

How to Inject Insulin:

a. Grasp the syringe so that the forefinger and thumb are around the top of syringe barrel.
b. Cleanse injection site.
c. Insert needle under skin or into muscle with the plunger and needle held at an angle similar to holding a pencil.
d. Inject insulin by pushing in plunger; withdraw needle quickly; with other hand press the area with zephiran sponge.
e. Wash reusable syringe and reusable needle with cold water and store in a clean container; if disposable syringe and needle have been used, damage them beyond repair before discarding.

Storage of Insulin:

a. Insulin should be kept in the refrigerator. Do not place it near the freezing unit.
b. Long-acting insulin bottle should be turned over gently two or three times immediately before using each day. Do not shake the bottle.
c. Check the expiration date on the box. If insulin is out of date, do not use it, but do ask for a replacement.

6: CAN THE PATIENT THROW AWAY
THE NEEDLE?

Understandably, some diabetics become impatient with the need for taking insulin. It does, of course, complicate daily activities and many a hope has been expressed for an insulin substitute which could be taken by mouth. These desires have stimulated through the years a laboratory search for chemicals capable of lowering the blood sugar, and at the same time have provided a fertile environment for quacks, charlatans, herb doctors, faith healers and peddlers of homemade remedies which are useless and directly or indirectly dangerous. What are the facts which should shape the attitudes and temper the hopes of the diabetic with respect to the daily injections of insulin?

1. Quackery

One of the most vicious characters in the world today is the medical quack who takes advantage of those who are ill.

Even normally sensible and staid citizens lose their sense of proportion and grasp at any promise which gives support to the hope for health for themselves or their loved ones. No suffering is grievous enough to arouse the pity of the quack. He says: "Come to me and I will cure your cancer," or "I have a magic herb which will make your diabetes go away." It is obvious to everyone but the victim that this is fakery because the formula is secret, its peddler refuses to have it tested by qualified scientists, and it is usually not offered free of charge. And yet the people flock even though there is no proof that the remedy provides any relief. Many patients have fallen prey to such appeals.

Dr. Charles E. Horton of Duke University points out, however, that not all quacks are dishonest: "In North Carolina we have been impressed with the genuine basic honesty of a few of the quack backwoods healers. It is their lack of education, not a desire to exploit the masses, that is the real cause of this evil." Nonetheless the sincerity of an honest though misguided quack does not make him any the less dangerous to the diabetic or to any other ailing patient. The fact that such a person is not under arrest and his actions appear to be condoned by the public authorities does not mean there is any merit in his program. This is merely an indication that it takes time to assemble evidence and to prosecute. In the interim the patient and his family will do well to keep in mind the definition of a quack as set up by a commission of the California Medical Association. This points out that a quack normally has one or more of the following characteristics:

1. His treatment is available only from himself.
2. His treatment bears his own name or that of a high-

sounding research organization.

3. His treatment is advertised.
4. He claims he is being persecuted by the "medical trusts."
5. His cured patients and greatest supporters have only his word for it that they had the disease in the first place.
6. He discourages or refuses consultations with reputable physicians.

Before the reader cries "Not me!" let's review the actual case history of Eileen M., born August 5, 1944, and her devoted mother. As a child of ten, Eileen had developed diabetes. The weight loss, weakness, and increased thirst which had appeared responded completely to treatment with diet and with insulin. All went well until the mother accepted the invitation of a neighbor to attend a religious meeting organized by a particularly persuasive female revivalist. This well-intentioned but overenthusiastic lady convinced Eileen's mother that Eileen could stop taking insulin and her diabetes would be cured. For a day or two all seemed well and then the child became desperately ill and would have died in coma if the mother had not relented at the last moment and brought her to the hospital.

The record is clear therefore as far as diabetic quackery and faith healing are concerned: it is extremely dangerous to succumb to the blandishments of such characters. But then, it is logical to ask if science has been any more successful in helping the diabetic to throw away the needle.

2. Science: oral anti-diabetic agents

In 1942 a Frenchman named Janbon reported at the 43rd Congress of Psychiatrists and Neurologists of France that a sulfa drug derivative, the chemical name of which was abbreviated to IPTD, produced a low blood-sugar level and even convulsions in patients. Janbon turned to a French physiologist, Auguste Loubatieres, for an explanation of this marked lowering of the blood-sugar levels. Loubatieres then embarked on a prolonged series of animal studies designed to identify the mechanism of this effect. Between 1942 and 1955 Loubatieres made many observations with IPTD and demonstrated the important fact that it lowered the level of blood sugar only in animals with a pancreas or a remnant thereof. He suggested therefore that the drug produced its effect either by stimulating a further secretion of insulin by the pancreas or by intensifying its effects.

As with many important findings, such as the classical work of Minkowski and Von Mehring showing that diabetes developed in animals deprived of the pancreas, the possible clinical usefulness of these findings in diabetes was not extensively explored by the original workers. In 1955 the hypoglycemic action of sulfa drugs and their derivatives was confirmed by a group of German scientists working in the famed pharmaceutical house of Boehringer and Sons. In seeking better agents amongst the sulfa drugs for the control of infections, they noted that one of the drugs produced lowering of the blood-sugar levels and convulsions in mice. The tests with this drug, tagged BZ55, were repeated in dogs with essentially the same results. Its relative safety was then established by the usual studies in animals. Trials were begun in diabetics only after tests in human volunteers. World-renowned specialists caring for diabetics, such as Bertram, undertook to test the drug in diabetic adults and children. They showed that BZ55 taken orally proved just as effective as insulin in some patients. For the first time in the history of mankind a way of treating diabetes without an injection was available, surpassing in efficiency the fondest hopes of even the most flagrant quacks. A related drug, D860, appeared just as effective. Extensive trials were then undertaken in many clinics and hospitals in Germany and the two drugs were introduced into the United States as Carbutamide   (BZ55) and Orinase   (D860). By the end of 1956 more than ten thousand diabetics had received Carbutamide   and four thousand had taken Orinase   for intervals up to one year in length. Much information has been accumulated about these two oral insulin substitutes. Thus, though many patients could stop taking insulin, others, particularly those with the childhood form of diabetes, responded but little if at all. Neither drug could replace insulin in treating diabetic acidosis and coma nor was the action intensive enough to regulate diabetes during an infection. There were indications that, in general, middle-aged patients with diabetes of recent onset responded better. As might be expected from our knowledge of the milder degrees of diabetes in overweight patients, such diabetics responded better to this treatment than the lean ones. However, in no one patient, young or old, fat or thin, with diabetes recently discovered or of life-long duration, could one be absolutely sure that these drugs would or would not work. Each individual had to be tested separately to determine his response, if any, to these insulin substitutes. Many found it possible to free themselves of the daily tedium of taking insulin simply by taking one, two, or three aspirin-sized tablets each day. And with this freedom came a bonus: less insulin shock. However, in October of 1956 the American firm which distributed Carbutamide   announced that some 5 per cent of the ten thousand diabetics on this drug had developed reactions which might have been caused by this insulin substitute. These included fever, skin rashes, and perhaps changes in the heart and liver. Very properly it was decided that since oral insulin substitutes were a convenience rather than an absolute need, distribution should be limited until further tests could be run. Tests with the other drug, Orinase (tolbutamide), and with related products such as Diabinese (chlorpropamide), Tolinase (tolazamide), Dymelor (acetohexamide) and Micronase (glyburide) have continued under the cautious direction of physicians. In the meantime, an entirely different oral anti-diabetic agent, phenformin or DBI, has come upon the scene.

Experience indicates that in many patients, but not all, treatment with a diet and one of these drugs provides satisfactory control of blood sugar. None of these agents is a true substitute for insulin, even though they do lower the blood sugar. Actually their beneficial action upon the regulation of diabetes always requires the presence of insulin.

None of the drugs should be used in any patient with a positive urine acetone test. If this test turns positive after previous negative tests, it is a sign that at that point the diabetes can no longer be controlled by the drug and insulin must be administered. This principle should never be violated if acidosis and coma are to be avoided.

Early in the 1970's, the results of a ten-year study of sulfonylureas and of phenformin in diabetic patients were reported by the University Group Diabetes Program (UGDP). The data suggested that use of these agents may in certain patients increase the risk of cardiac deaths. The Food and Drug Administration and other agencies have informed your physician of these findings and he takes all of these facts into account in guiding your treatment.

3. Sulfonylurea and phenformin therapy

There are two classes of oral anti-diabetic agents in current use throughout most of the world—the sulfonylureas and the biguanides. In the USA only the sulfonylureas are available, following the withdrawal of phenformin, a biguanide, by the Food and Drug Agency. On the European continent two biguanides, metformin and buformin, are prescribed. The sulfonylureas and biguanides differ in chemical structure and produce their effects through entirely different mechanisms.

The sulfonylureas are prescribed for diabetic persons whose pancreas is still capable of secreting insulin, viz. those with Stage III or IV non-insulin-dependent diabetes. In such individuals, the sulfonylureas increase the manufacture and release of insulin in response to food and perhaps decrease the secretion of glucagon, a pancreatic hormone which raises blood sugar levels. The sulfonylureas also affect tissues other than the pancreas but these are not significant from the viewpoint of diabetes control.

Phenformin on the other hand acts through a different mechanism. It does not increase the insulin supplies but it does accelerate the use of glucose provided that glucose is already being used. In other words, if the person has enough insulin of his own or enough has been given to him and sugar is being metabolized, then phenformin increases the rate at which this occurs. Phenformin also has a second action: it controls the rate at which food is absorbed and thereby prevents overloading of the disposal mechanisms.

In those diabetic individuals who have ketone bodies in the urine or in the blood, sulfonylureas or phenformin will not work to lower the sugar level. The ketone bodies usually indicate that the ability of the pancreas to manufacture and to release insulin is either greatly reduced or totally absent. The sulfonylureas cannot be expected to increase the secretion of insulin sufficiently to permit control of the diabetes and phenformin will not accelerate the use of glucose. In other words, persons with diabetes and ketone bodies in the urine, or a history of diabetic ketosis, acidosis, or coma usually have a marked insulin-deficiency and are (or have been) in Stage V, VI, or VII of diabetes. Such insulin deficiency has to be treated with injected insulin and cannot be treated with sulfonylureas alone or with phenformin alone.

In those patients who have Stage III or IV diabetes and hence by definition possess considerable residual ability to secrete insulin, one of the sulfonylureas or phenformin or both can often provide highly satisfactory control of the diabetes. Four preparations of sulfonylurea are available on the American market.

Of the sulfonylureas Orinase or tolbutamide has the shortest (4–5 hours), and Diabinese or chlorpropamide has the longest duration of action (24+ hours), The insulin releasing and other effects of Dymelor or acetohexamide and of Tolinase or tolazamide are of intermediate duration (12 to 18 hours). Each of the sulfonylureas is taken in the morning just before breakfast. However, because of its short duration of action, additional Orinase may be taken with either one or both of the other meals, and additional Dymelor or Tolinase may be prescribed for the evening meal.

In Europe and elsewhere, Glyburide (glibenclamide) is in wide use. Its effect lasts several hours.

Phenformin is taken with or after meals one to three times daily.

Neither the biguanides nor the sulfonylureas replace diet

control in the management of diabetes. Both are to be used only with a diabetic meal program. In the usual sequence of treatment of newly discovered diabetes in Stage III or IV the diet is changed to reduce starches or sugars and, if the patient is overweight, the total calories are reduced as well. If such a program does control the blood as well as the urine sugar adequately, then no additional treatment is needed. In other words, the load of starches and sugars and of calories is cut to the point where the ability of the body to use sugar, though reduced, again becomes adequate to meet the daily needs. If such restriction of sugars and of starches and of calories does not control the blood and urine sugar, then one of the oral anti-diabetic agents in the sulfonylurea group or a biguanide is prescribed.

In some instances the physician may prescribe both a sulfonylurea and a biguanide since their mechanisms of action are different and therefore additive.

No additional benefit is to be expected from giving two different sulfonylureas at one time. However, the physician may substitute one sulfonylurea for another in the hope of obtaining an improved insulin response.

Again, it should be emphasized that the appearance of ketone bodies in the urine during trials of diet, sulfonylurea, or a biguanide is a signal for an instantaneous shift to insulin to control the diabetes. When such a shift is carried out during ketonuria, the sulfonylurea or biguanide is discontinued.

The oral anti-diabetic agents are remarkably safe drugs, but they can produce side reactions or toxic effects. Thus, episodes of low blood sugar (hypoglycemia) may occur in patients with diabetes who are receiving one or the other of the sulfonylureas. As one might expect, these are most common in those persons taking the longest or the longer-acting of the sulfonylureas but hypoglycemia may also develop during Orinase (tolbutamide) treatment. Low blood sugars never or almost never occur with a biguanide as the sole drug treatment.

The sulfonylureas may rarely produce skin rashes, drug fever, or gastrointestinal upsets. They can also lower thyroid function.

The biguanides may produce gastrointestinal distress of various types, i.e. a metallic taste, abdominal discomfort, diarrhea, etc., particularly if the ordinary tablets are used. Such complaints were much less frequent when DBI-TD (Timed Disintegration) capsules of phenformin were used.

Some physicians believe that phenformin is a frequent cause of a "Lactic Acidosis Syndrome." However, most of the time when lactic acidosis does appear in either a diabetic or non-diabetic person it is caused by deficient oxygenation of the tissues from causes other than phenformin. It is true that in diabetic persons with kidney failure, lactic acidosis is more apt to occur during phenformin treatment. However, phenformin should not be used in kidney failure or any other serious illness including liver disease, heart failure, bleeding from the gut, alcoholism, etc.

This problem of lactic acidosis has led to the withdrawal of phenformin from the U.S. market.

7 : WHAT MAKES DIABETES WORSE?

There are patients who on diet alone or with an anti-diabetic agent and/or insulin are gratifyingly free of high blood-sugar levels and show satisfactory urine tests day in and day out. In most patients, however, a variety of factors, recognized and unrecognized, influence the day-to-day regulation. The former include exercise, infections, menstrual periods, menopause, emotional upsets, variations in the diet, "juggling" of the insulin dosage, insulin shock, and the rare disorders of endocrine glands such as the thyroid, pituitary, adrenal, etc. which occasionally affect the diabetic.

1. Physical inactivity

Adults or children who engage in extra physical exertion during a week of work or of vacation may be less active on Saturday or Sunday. Under this circumstance it is not unusual for them to find that the urine sugar increases over the weekend. This is quite understandable since we know that exercise accelerates the use of carbohydrate and other foods by the body. As a matter of fact, with extensive exercising the diabetic on insulin can even bring on an insulin shock. The best way to compensate for these fluctuations in physical activity is to increase the food intake in the between-meal feedings on days when exertion is heavy. The alternative possibility of changing insulin dosage should be employed only if the extra food proves to be an insufficient measure.

2. Infections

Most patients have learned from experience that an ordinary cold, sore throat, stomach upset of the influenzal type, infection of the urine, etc., makes their diabetes worse. Part of this may be related to the decrease in activity which illness of any kind tends to bring about. This is not the entire explanation, however, since the loss of regulation is noted even when the patient continues to work or go to school. It is probable that during such an infection either anti-insulin factors are released, the production of sugar in the body is increased, or both. We know, for example, that illness increases the activity of the outer part of the adrenal gland (see section 4 of this chapter and the Appendix). The hormones that are thereby released to the blood stream in increased amounts cancel in part the effectiveness of insulin in increasing the use of glucose and at the same time increase the manufacture of new sugar by the tissues. There may well be other as yet unidentified factors liberated by the infecting virus or bacteria or by tissues in response to these invaders which have similar effects. It is also possible that during an infection insulin is destroyed more rapidly.

3. Role of menstrual periods, birth control pills, menopause

Girls and women with diabetes recognize that just before the monthly period the sugar increases in the urine and acetone may appear even when they continue their usual program of diabetic control. Though the changes in physical activity, in dietary habits, and in mood which accompany menstruation may play a role, there is also a real hormonal basis for this. Studies in animals and observations in humans have demonstrated that increases in female sex hormones in the small amounts which occur during menstruation do increase the tendency to diabetes or make it worse if it is already present. This often requires a temporary increase in insulin dosage.

Birth control pills may have an adverse effect on diabetes, but this is unusual. Also, the changes are usually minor and disappear when the medication is discontinued.

There are, however, women who develop diabetes at the change of life, i.e., at menopause, when one might expect the chances of diabetes to be less because of decreased sex hormone production. This presumably means that other factors are more important such as advancing age, a tendency to becoming overweight, a decrease in physical activity, or other unidentified changes in hormones and tissues.

4. Effect of emotions in diabetic regulation

In the course of the menstrual cycle a mild degree of emotional depression is not at all unusual. As already suggested, perhaps this plays a role in the worsening of diabetic control observed at that time. Certainly physicians are quite aware of the marked effects of emotional upsets upon the body chemistry in general and upon the metabolism of foodstuffs and of sugar in particular. There have been many observations of children and of adults whose diabetes becomes more severe or actual acidosis develops following a disturbing event in school or at work, a conflict with friends or family, an emotional shock, etc. It is probable that the discharge of adrenalin by the inner part of the adrenal gland, the medulla, which accompanies such upsets (an observation made many years ago by the famed physiologist Walter B. Cannon as described in his book, *Bodily Changes in Pain, Hunger, Fear and Rage,* published by D. Appleton and Co., New York, 2nd Ed., 1929), plays a role. Adrenalin stops insulin secretion, releases sugar from the liver and muscles, and may partially block its use by the tissues. Also, it is likely that a release of steroid hormones by the outer part of the adrenal, the cortex, which is known to occur in stressful situations, is a factor. As indicated in section 2 of this chapter, these steroids block the blood-sugar-lowering effect of insulin and at the same time increase the new formation of sugar. It is important to recognize the role of emotions upon diabetic regulation because with insight such episodes will be less disturbing and provision in the form of extra insulin and readjustments in the daily program can be made to compensate for them.

5. Loss of control following irregularities of diet and of insulin administration

In all these specific examples of factors such as decreased activity, infection, menstrual changes, and emotional disturbances which affect diabetic regulation, one must keep in mind the possible role of altered food intake and variable insulin administration. Obviously, if an upset stomach or abdominal discomfort results in a loss of appetite and interferes with the eating of regular meals, the orderly metabolism of the body is altered. The body has to manufacture glucose from its tissues and to call forth the stores of fat to meet energy requirements. It is easy to understand how under these circumstances the levels of sugar in blood and urine and the production of ketone bodies would be raised. Similarly, if a patient overeats because an emotional upset causes a gnawing discomfort which can be relieved by food, it is logical to find the sugar increased. Actually, there are patients who may overeat to arouse the solicitude, concern, worry or anger of their families despite the fact that in this process they may be inflicting harm on themselves. The human organism is a mass of complicated interrelationships and major consequences may result from simple beginnings. If one keeps this fact in mind it will be easier to understand some of the so-called spontaneous day-to-day changes in the intensity of the diabetes.

It is easy to see why altering the insulin dosage away from the ideal amount may adversely affect diabetes. If a patient requires a certain amount of insulin each day, decreasing the dosage without good indication for such a move will obviously increase blood and urine sugar and the ketone levels. Yet many patients do exactly this when for some reason they cannot eat their full diet. They reason that the less they eat the less the insulin need. They forget, however, two extremely important facts: 1) the body still needs insulin even when all food is cut off because there are some stores of carbohydrate in the body and because the tissues, especially the cells of the liver, continue to produce glucose from body protein and other materials; and 2) the illness, emotional upset, or other factor which interferes with eating may at the same time raise the insulin requirement. The patient is right, however, in being concerned about a possible insulin shock when the usual dietary habits are interrupted. It may be necessary to reduce the dosage to prevent such shocking but the tests of urine for sugar and for acetone should serve as guides in such adjustments. Practically never is it reasonable to omit the insulin entirely.

6. Insulin shock as an aggravator of diabetes

Insulin shock, recognized or unrecognized, complicates regulation and makes the diabetes worse. Of course, such insulin shocking lowers the blood sugar and this hypoglycemia in turn evokes a rise in hormones which combat low blood-sugar levels. The latter include growth hormone, glucagon, adrenalin, and cortisol which then make the diabetes more severe. At times the insulin shocking is not recognized but these anti-insulin factors nonetheless rise and the dosage of insulin is increased rather than decreased. Perhaps the best way of illustrating this is to point out that from time to time doctors see patients who have progressively increased their dosage above the original requirement by repeated shocking. This may occur at night when the patient is asleep and there may be no distinct indication of such shocking as far as the patient is concerned. As pointed out in Chapter 10, which deals with insulin shock, he may just awaken feeling tired, or with a headache. On the other hand the insulin shocks may be quite clear-cut and be recognized by the patient. Such repeated shocking tends to make the diabetes worse, increases the urine sugar, and leads the patient to raise the insulin dosage further. The patient is caught in a vicious circle. This has been called the Somogyi effect after the physician who first described it. At this point the patient becomes frantic because despite evidences of too large an insulin dosage the urine sugar remains high. Under these circumstances, or whenever the insulin requirements have changed markedly, the patient should consult the physician who will seek out factors known to produce such variations.

7. Diabetes and disorders of the hormone-producing glands

It has already been pointed out that one of the endocrine glands, the ovary, may in the course of its normal function aggravate the severity of diabetes. Another gland, the adrenal, may do the same as its two parts, the medulla and cortex, respond to stressful situations. Insofar as the other endocrines are concerned, diabetes may rarely be the result of a disturbance of a hormone-producing gland such as the pituitary, or thyroid, but previously present diabetes may be made worse by disorders of these organs. This is such a comparatively rare occurrence that it is of no importance in the day-to-day regulation of diabetes.

Glucagon, the blood-sugar-raising hormone of the alpha cells of the pancreas, may be inappropriately high or inappropriately low in diabetes.

For practical purposes, therefore, the patient who is encountering difficulty in achieving smooth control should quickly ask whether this could be the result of varying physical activity or an obvious or hidden infection, is it cyclic and perhaps related to menstrual periods, is there an emotional problem present, might it be explained by irregularities of diet or of insulin dosage, or by obvious or undetected insulin shock? Having gone through such a check list, the patient will have considered all of the ordinary reasons for fluctuations in the diabetic control and will in all probability recognize that one or more of them are contributing to the problem. Resolution of the difficulty often requires a dual responsibility, that of the doctor and of the patient, but it is a realistic and obviously desirable goal.

8 : CAN DIABETES BE CURED?

The first sigh of relief breathed after learning that the wastage of flesh and the loss of strength which may have been troubling a patient or his family was the result of diabetes and not some dreaded disease is quickly followed by the query: "Doctor, can diabetes be cured?" Though this characteristic and very human question could be disposed of promptly and effectively by a categorical "No," this would be an incomplete answer. It has already been pointed out that not all newly diagnosed patients are alike: some have major symptoms which will require intensive treatment with diet and insulin before relief is obtained and health is restored, while others learn of the presence of diabetes during a routine physical examination or pre-insurance check-up. However, not only does diabetes vary in severity from individual to individual but great variations may be occasionally seen in the same person. In the preceding chapter factors known to increase the intensity of diabetes have been discussed. When and under what circumstances can one expect a decrease in the severity of diabetes and may this ever be great enough to remove any and all vestiges of it?

1. Conditions under which diabetes may be expected to become less severe

A. IN INDIVIDUALS WHO ARE OVERWEIGHT AT THE ONSET OF DIABETES

Most grossly overweight patients can expect to reduce their insulin dosage or eliminate it entirely if they follow a low-calorie reducing diet. They must lose a sufficient amount of weight to achieve and hold this goal. This is not a new observation. First, it will be recalled from Chapter 4 that the early studies of Doctors Allen, Stillman and Fitz, in the pre-insulin era, demonstrated that total starvation of patients for a week or longer decreased the levels of sugar in urine and in blood. Such starvation reduced the foodstuffs to, or closer to, the point where the cells, though handicapped by insulin lack, could handle the load summoned from the tissues for the maintenance of life. Second, as body size and the mass of living tissue decrease, less energy is necessary to maintain body temperature, to pump blood, and to replace aging units in the normal wear and tear of living. This makes it possible to meet the energy demands of the body with a lesser amount of food. Under these conditons a point is often reached at which the diminished insulin-producing and food-utilizing capacities again prove adequate.

It is no longer usual to prescribe complete starvation for this purpose. Rather the dietary intake is adjusted downward with careful provision for a sufficient amount of the necessary protein and enough carbohydrate to avoid the undesirable chemical effects of starvation. The tissues then draw upon fat stores to make up the balance of needed energy and the body weight falls.

It should be obvious that this program is not a 14-day "banana and skim milk" or any other dietary fad but rather a permanent way of life. Increasing the intake of food and the regaining of body weight will again bring back the diabetes with all of its manifestations. In other words, the diabetes is still present. It has not disappeared but if overweight is corrected it remains under virtually perfect control.

B. IN PATIENTS WHO RECOVER FROM AN INFECTION, BECOME ACTIVE AFTER A PERIOD IN BED, ARE RELIEVED OF EMOTIONAL PROBLEMS, OR IN WHOM UNRECOGNIZED INSULIN SHOCKING IS CORRECTED

It is logical to expect that if "a straw can break a camel's back," removing the added burden should be beneficial. The subsidence of an acute "cold" or a sore throat, the successful treatment of an infection of the ear, of the urine, or of any organ or system, removes the straw that makes the diabetes worse. The same is true of the other factors known to increase the severity of diabetes. If it so happens that the diabetes is fundamentally mild, one can expect it to return to this same state once the aggravating factors are removed.

C. DIABETES BECOMES MILDER WHEN ABNORMAL OVERACTIVITY OF
THE PITUITARY, THYROID OR THE ADRENAL GLAND IS CORRECTED

In the preceding chapter it was pointed out that abnormal overactivity of any of these three glands makes diabetes worse. In terms of the total diabetic population such overactivity arising spontaneously is a rare event; all of these conditions represent major and unusual disturbances of these glands of internal secretion. The exact details of the symptoms and signs of the overactivity of each of these glands are presented in the Appendix and need not concern us here save to state that they can be detected by suitable physical and laboratory examinations. A decrease in the severity of the diabetes can be expected with appropriate treatment should any one of these conditons develop.

2. Real "cures" in diabetes

A complete disappearance of diabetes is an extremely uncommon occurrence. The fundamental problem in diabetes is a shortage of insulin or insulin action and so far there has been no cure for this deficiency except continued treatment. From the viewpoint of insulin reserve, there are a number of borderline individuals present in all of the age groups of our population. A crucial infection in such children or adults may precipitate an obvious diabetes which may then disappear as the infection subsides. In all of the modern-day literature there are only a few such instances recorded in children. The rate is also low in adults, if one excludes the temporary diabetic-like state produced by cortisone, ACTH, or other drug treatment.

For all practical purposes, therefore, diabetes once it

appears persists for the life of the individual even though the aggravating factors such as infection, inactivity, emotional upset, etc., are removed. It is true, however, that with advancing years elderly diabetics may require less insulin. It has also been noted that following two or more pregnancies, the insulin requirement may be less and that the same change may occur in some patients with diabetes who develop certain kidney complications.

9 : ACIDOSIS AND COMA

In the days before insulin, acidosis or coma was an extremely serious complication of diabetes. It often brought death and a welcome release from the misery of a life of privation, weakness, and starvation to many adults and to almost all children with diabetes.

1. The risks of acidosis and coma today

Contrast this truly frightening prospect with the facts of today: with proper care it is possible to have diabetes for an entire lifetime and never develop acidosis or coma. If acidosis or coma does occur and prompt and proper care is provided, it turns out to be a mere event in the life of a diabetic. This is not to say, however, that acidosis or coma is no longer a hazard for diabetics nor that it need not be prevented. It is true that during a single decade we treated more than two hundred children with acidosis and coma (*American Journal of Diseases of Children,* Vol. 93, pages 341-56, 1957) without the loss of a single diabetic previously under our care, and the record is equally good in many other clinics. We have, however, seen coma end fatally in five diabetic children in this period. Without exception this has occurred in *previously undiagnosed* diabetics who had been in acidosis or coma for many hours or days, and in whom treatment was not prompt because of delays in diagnosis and in transportation to a qualified treatment center. These irreversible cases make up only 2 per cent of our total group of acidosis and coma in children, but even these can be prevented or treated successfully with early diagnosis and care. In the adult members of our diabetic population the hazards are greater, chiefly because older people often have complicating diseases of the heart, kidney, brain and other organs and because delay in seeking attention may be very great indeed in the case of patients who live alone and become ill. And yet with excellent guidance and prompt and adequate care, the risk in adults can be reduced, as it has been in the justifiably famous Joslin Clinic, to levels as low as those prevailing in the younger population.

2. Who may develop diabetic acidosis-coma?

If prevention is the key, under what conditions is acidosis or coma especially apt to occur? If early treatment is important, what are the very first signs to be looked for? From our records and the experience of many other clinics it is amply clear that the previously undiagnosed and unrecognized patient is especially liable to develop acidosis or coma. Fortunately, diabetes which reaches this stage of complication is quite obvious. It screams for recognition for weeks or months with symptoms of increased thirst, increased passage of urine, weight loss (often in the face of increased appetite), generalized weakness, irritation of the external genitals in females and the other manifestations summarized in Chapter 3. Hence, hoping that symtoms of diabetes will quietly go away by calling them a "cold in the kidneys" or an attack of "flu" is a certain invitation to trouble. It is natural to behave this way if one has previously enjoyed a lifetime of good health, and so dangerous in the case of diabetes! Early recognition of the presence of diabetes by prompt consultation with a physician or clinic for examination of the urine and blood sugar whenever suggestive symptoms appear, and periodic health checks which include at least a urine analysis and a blood sugar determination, especially two hours after a meal, are the only ways in which unnecessary delays can be avoided.

3. Early detection of diabetes as a prevention of acidosis-coma

In the case of those of us who have no symptoms whatsoever, who should be especially careful in watching for the possible appearance of diabetes? The answer is simple: all those who are overweight and any who come from a family with a history of diabetes or of giving birth to large babies.

Under what conditons might an individual develop diabetic symptoms? The experience on this point is quite clear. Infections, major or minor, including "colds" among the latter, and abdominal ailments such as inflammation of the gall bladder or of the pancreas are especially prone to bring out a previously dormant diabetes, or a tendency thereto. However, diabetes has been detected for the first time following a fracture or other illness with enforced rest in bed, in connection with an emotional shock or a mental illness, or even after an ordinarily inconsequential procedure such as vaccination against smallpox. The experience in our clinic in this regard is shown in table II.

Exactly the same events may precede acidosis or coma in the previously diagnosed patient save that an additional one may be present in some patients: insulin shocking may set off a train of events leading to this complication.

TABLE II

Antecedent events in 191 episodes of acidosis and coma in children

	*Per Cent of Patients**
Previously undiagnosed	31
Poor control	42
Insulin omission	20
Insulin shock	6
Infection	61
Emotional upset	20

* In some patients several of the above causes were present.

4. First signs

Acidosis and coma are almost always preceded by acute or chronic signs of a lack or loss of diabetic regulation, i.e., increased passage of urine during the day and night and increased thirst and consumption of water. Urine analyses show ketone bodies and sugar, usually to the point of an orange-red test, i.e., 4+, if Benedict's solution is used. Acetone may be detected on the breath as a sweetish odor. At this time or earlier the patient usually feels ill, loses interest in eating, and begins to vomit any fluids or food which may be taken. The vomiting may be repeated and severe enough to produce abdominal pain. At this point the patient is said to be in keto-acidosis or in acidosis (these terms are explained below). The face often becomes flushed and the breathing becomes rapid. Later, "air hunger" may develop with deep as well as rapid respirations, and stupor or unconsciousness may set in. When the latter stage is reached, coma is said to be present. The actual occurrence of these symptoms and signs in a group of some four hundred of our diabetic children and adults is shown in table III.

Table III

*Symptoms and signs in acidosis and coma
in children and adults*

Symptoms and Signs	Per Cent of Children* (191 episodes)	Per Cent of Adults** (188 episodes)
Vomiting	79	71
Abdominal pain	39	—
Loss of consciousness	8	24
Rapid breathing	71	100
Low blood pressure	0	32

*American Journal of Diseases of Children, Vol. 93: pp. 341-56, 1957.

**Yale Journal of Biology and Medicine, Vol. 18: pp. 405-17, 1946.

5. When should the patient and the family become concerned about the possibility of acidosis and coma?

The answer to this question is simple: whenever diabetes becomes uncontrolled, whenever the symptoms or signs which have been described appear, and *especially whenever the patient begins to vomit.* The doctor should be consulted immediately and, if there is any delay in communicating with him, the patient should be taken to the emergency room of the nearest hospital with facilities adequate for the care of diabetes. The need for haste becomes all the more urgent if air hunger or unconsciousness appears. However, even in the advanced case the doctor should be called, since he may wish to recommend that insulin treatment be started in the home before taking the patient to the hospital.

6. What is the chemical disturbance in diabetic acidosis and coma?

When a shortage of insulin is present because of diabetes and particularly when infection, inactivity, or an emotional disturbance makes this lack even more pronounced, sugar cannot be used to a normal degree and the body begins to rely more and more on fat for the energy necessary for the beating of the heart, the process of breathing, and the many other activities of the cells. This shift to fat as a fuel is possible because the tissues can extract energy from it even when a shortage of insulin is present. In summoning forth the fat stored in the tissues, more appears than can be used. The acids in this fat (appropriately called fatty acids) are broken down into ketone bodies (small fatty acids called beta hydroxybutyric and aceto-acetic and a product of the latter, acetone) which accumulate in the body fluids and spill over in the urine. The ketone bodies upset the delicate hydrogen ion space balance in the body and cause an acidosis. As acidosis progresses the body tries to compensate for this by blowing off carbonic acid through the lungs, and hence the rapid and deep breathing.

The level of sugar rises because in the face of an insulin shortage glucose cannot be used by cells at a normal rate. At the same time the body, especially the liver, continues to make new sugar from proteins and from glycerol. As the level rises sugar spills into the urine and increases the formation and flow of urine, thereby decreasing the body water and producing thirst. At the same time important minerals are also lost in the urine, including the two chief ones in body fluids, sodium and potassium. The net effect is a deficit of body water and of minerals. As this becomes more pronounced the efficiency of the circulation and the clarity of the mind may become impaired. This, however, is not the sole cause of the loss of consciousness which may occur, and a completely satisfactory explanation for this manifestation of acidosis and coma is still lacking.

7. How acidosis and coma are treated

The physician has two major jobs before him: he must restore the use of sugar back to normal, and he must correct the disturbances of the body fluids, that is, the acidosis, the deficits of water and minerals, and their consequences.

The early phase of the treatment of an acidosis or coma is a demanding moment. Blood is drawn, small or large amounts of insulin are injected (often some is given by vein to hasten its action), and mixtures of sodium and other minerals and, at times, plasma or plasma substitutes are put into the veins. When the laboratory results are available, and especially as the patient begins to respond, the prescription is modified to include sugar * and potassium while insulin administration and the other measures are continued. As consciousness returns and the air hunger disappears, the patient is offered sips of water, broth, or tea with sugar. Ultimately the injection of solutions is discontinued and the patient returns to a normal diabetic diet. It may take the better part of the day or longer to complete the recovery and several days to convalesce. There are no permanent ill effects. Before the patient's discharge from the hospital, the cause of the coma is sought and the lesson thereby learned applied to prevention of further such episodes. As indicated earlier, acidosis and coma are not inevitable complications of diabetes. Most patients never experience them because they apply preventive measures which consist of appropriate adjustments in insulin dosage during infections, other illnesses, periods of inactivity, emotional upset or insulin shocking.

* This seems contradictory since the blood sugar is already high. Actually, the total amount of sugar in the body fluids is small; once insulin starts to work the level drops sharply and glucose has to be given to permit insulin to continue its beneficial action with safety.

10 : INSULIN SHOCK, ACIDOSIS-COMA, AND OTHER CAUSES OF STUPOR OR LOSS OF CONSCIOUSNESS IN DIABETES

The diabetic may become stuporous, unresponsive, or unconscious because of diabetic acidosis-coma or from insulin shock. These are the two most common causes, but coma can develop for other reasons unrelated or related to the diabetes. Thus, it may be incidental, as with brain injury or poisoning, or may result from a shortage of oxygen in the tissues (lactic acidosis) or very high levels of sugar or sodium in the blood (hypersomolar coma). It is important to be aware of these alternative possibilities, however, so that valuable time is not lost in treating the diabetic for acidosis-coma or insulin shock when the patient should be receiving other specialized attention.

1.   Differentiation of acidosis-coma and insulin shock

In the preceding chapter it has been pointed out that acidosis-coma is a complication of unregulated or inadequately regulated diabetes. Therefore, to establish this as the cause of unconsciousness in a patient, one should obtain an antecedent history of increased thirst and increased volumes of urine with large amounts of sugar and acetone. There may be other symptoms of uncontrolled diabetes such as weight loss, fatigability, genital irritation in the female, etc. Loss of consciousness in acidosis-coma is gradual rather than abrupt and very often is preceded by loss of appetite and vomiting and by deep breathing of the air-hunger type. The episode is usually ushered in by a cold or other respiratory infection, failure to take insulin, an emotional upset, or may even follow a severe insulin shock. Upon examination, such a diabetic has dry lips, a flushed face, and rapid deep breathing in addition to being unresponsive. Sweating is usually not present. Benedict's or similar tests of the urine for sugar show 4+, i.e., orange-red, reduction, and acetone and other ketones are present in large amounts. One must be sure, however, that the urine that is obtained for examination is representative of the conditions existing at that moment and not a confusing residue from an earlier period. The blood sugar is almost always greatly elevated. The carbon dioxide in serum is decreased, largely because of the accumulation of ketone bodies cited above.

In insulin shock or hypoglycemia, on the other hand, the history is quite different. The onset of unconsciousness is usually quite sudden in a patient previously well and normally responsive. The indices of diabetic control before this event are often satisfactory, though it is of course possible to have insulin shock occurring in a poorly regulated diabetic. The family may give a history of excessive exercise, omission of a meal, or of failure to adjust insulin dosage in accord with results of urine tests. The onset of insulin shock may be so rapid that the patient may become aware of such an event only when he recovers consciousness. Also in the case of insulin shocks occurring during sleep there may be no warning symptoms, but again the presence of headaches and peculiar sensations on awakening may be the clue to insulin shocking. In most patients, however, insulin shock is ushered in by a feeling of nervousness and apprehension and, if the patient is on short-acting insulin, is often accompanied by sweating. Visual disturbances may be present. If these symptoms are not followed by prompt administration of sugar or food the patient progresses into insulin shock and may develop twitching or convulsions. At examination the patient is unconscious but not overbreathing. Signs of dehydration are not present. Sweating may be evident. The urine examination reveals but little sugar, or none at all, if care is taken to obtain a freshly formed and freshly passed specimen. If acetone or other ketone bodies are present, it is only in trace amounts. Blood-sugar levels are low if the sample is drawn during the insulin shock. If this is delayed, the level may become normal as the liver pours out glucose in response to the low blood sugar, but it will not be high as it is in acidosis or coma. Also, hypoglycemia may be relative, i.e. a sudden drop from 300 to 75 mg%.

2. Overlap of manifestations of diabetic acidosis-coma and insulin shock

One should not be left with the impression that differentiation of the three chief causes of unconsciousness in the diabetic is always easy. In table IV the similarities and differences have been listed.

TABLE IV

Some similarities and differences in loss of consciousness in the diabetic occurring for one of several reasons

	Acidosis-Coma	Insulin Shock	Other Causes
History of poor regulation	Yes	Maybe	Not necessary
Antecedent infecness, or emotional upset	Often	Usually no	Not necessary
Omission or decrease in insulin	Frequent	No	No
Omission of food	Frequent	Frequent	No
Vomiting	Frequent	No	No
Strenuous exercise	No	Yes	Usually not
Stupor or coma	Present	Present	Present
Deep, rapid and regular breathing	Yes	No, shallow	No, but may get irregular breathing $\bar{c}$ cerebral disease

	Acidosis-Coma	Insulin Shock	Other Causes
Convulsions	No	Maybe	Maybe $\bar{c}$ cerebral disease
Sweating	Usually no	May be present, but not with long-acting insulin	Maybe
Urine sugar	High	Low or absent if recent urine is obtained	Not remarkable
Urine ketone bodies	Yes	Usually not but depends on previous regulation	Usually not but depends on previous regulation
Blood sugar	High	Low but may be normal if measured long after shock	Not high nor low

3. Treatment of insulin shock

Once it has been established that the patient is in insulin shock, glucose or other sugars should be administered. If the patient can swallow, this can be in the form of fruit juices with or without added sugar. If the patient cannot swallow, fluids should not be given since they will produce choking spells or interfere with breathing. Under these circumstances concentrated glucose is injected into the vein by the physician at home or in the emergency room of the hospital. Glucagon or adrenalin, which release sugar stored as glycogen in the liver and in other ways correct the low blood sugar, may be administered, though this is not the treatment of first choice. It should be kept in mind that not all patients respond promptly. The author has seen patients in such deep shock that it has taken hours for recovery. Though this is unusual, it is mentioned so that uncertainty about the accuracy of the diagnosis does not arise simply because the patient does not respond immediately after the administration of sugar.

However, the treatment should not be considered finished with recovery of consciousness. The cause should be ferreted out and every attempt made to prevent a recurrence. Is the patient receiving too much insulin, did he fail to take his diet, were in-between-meal feedings omitted, did the patient exercise heavily without anticipating the need for an extra intake of food? Careful search should be made for undetected shocking during the night. The only evidence of this may be thrashing about in bed, biting the tongue, or awakening in the morning with a headache, peculiar sensations in the extremities, or a "hung-over" feeling. The diet and insulin should then be adjusted to prevent shocking, keeping in mind that the goal of diabetic regulation is a normal blood sugar, not an abnormally low blood sugar. As much as we wish to keep the urine sugar free, clear tests twenty-four hours a day in a patient on insulin should be viewed as possible indications that such a person may be receiving too much insulin and might be on the verge of shock.

In some patients special problems may be responsible for the shocking. Thus in patients who cannot empty their bladder of urine completely, the urine tests may produce a false sense of security because they contain sugar passed many hours earlier. Also, in pregnancy milk sugar which reduces Benedict's solution and Clinitest® tablets (but not Tes-Tape® or Glucostix®) may be confused with glucose, and the insulin dosage raised unnecessarily. In patients on penicillin or on aspirin-like drugs false positive test may be obtained and similar mistakes made. Finally there are a few patients who spill sugars other than glucose, such as fruit sugar (fructose), galactose, etc., which confuse the picture.

4. Dangers of insulin shock

Insulin shock should not be taken lightly even though it is usually readily corrected. It may lead to brain injury and permanent damage. No doctor wishes to achieve diabetic control in the sense of normal blood sugars and urines free of sugar if the price is to be insulin shocking.

5. Wise precautions in diabetes

All patients should have a wrist or neck tag and a wallet card (see sample) stating he or she has diabetes, carry several lumps of sugar to offset impending shock, and adjust insulin or oral medication in accord with the doctor's advice if shocking has occurred. However, under no circumstances should insulin be discontinued entirely, because this will bring on acidosis-coma in insulin-dependent diabetes.

As with other complications of diabetes there are many patients who take insulin all of their lives and never experience an insulin shock. This is usually true of the well-controlled patient whose intake of food day in and day out is regular, and who makes the necessary adjustments in insulin dosage in accord with the results of regular urine testing. This is particularly essential when insulin require-ments decrease during recovery from an illness or as a consequence of extra physical activity. Similar adjustments should be made in the rare instances of insulin shock produced by the oral anti-diabetic agents. A regular program of between-meal feedings even in a sedentary patient, with additional intake of food after heavy exercise, is particularly helpful in preventing insulin shocks and achieving smooth control of the diabetes.

SAMPLE CARD FOR PATIENTS

FRONT

I HAVE DIABETES

If I am found unconscious or behaving abnormally, my condition may be the result of an overdose of insulin.

please see other side

BACK

please see other side

I have diabetes. Place sugar or candy in my mouth if I can swallow and call my physician or send me immediately to a hospital.

NAME ....

ADDRESS ....

PHYSICIAN'S NAME ....

ADDRESS ....

TELEPHONE ....

Identification card to be carried by the patient. Cards of this type may be obtained from the American Diabetes Association, Inc. 600 Fifth Avenue, New York, New York 10020, from your physician, or from your pharmacist.

11 : SPECIAL PROBLEMS IN DIABETES

Before the days of insulin it was accepted that almost all children and as many as 60 per cent of adults with diabetes were destined to die in coma. The advent of insulin and the more complete understanding of the chemical and related disturbances which characterize diabetic acidosis have reduced the mortality in children and adults from this cause to the vanishing point, provided, as has been pointed out in Chapter 9, that the patient, the physician, and the hospital succeed (and this really is a reasonable and attainable goal) in applying these principles in each particular case. The patient and his family are key links in this chain of success: they must and can, as the records clearly prove, acquire as complete an understanding as possible of the factors which precipitate acidosis and avoid or compensate for them. Alerted to the key signs and symptoms, the patient seeks the guidance of the physician and of the hospital at the precise point which separates any of the acceptable nonalarming day-to-day fluctuations in the diabetic regulation from the developments which usher in acidosis. At that moment the doctor and the hospital enter the picture with the highly effective treatment tools now available: the need for large or small amounts of insulin can be met quickly. The inability to drink and eat to provide the needed water, minerals and energy foods and the deficits that are incurred during the period of inadequate diabetic regulation can be overcome by injection of suitable fluids into the vein and into tissues. Any ill effects that have resulted from the shortage of insulin and the losses of body fluids and minerals can be canceled by appropriate treatment. The result: another instance of acidosis-coma is merely an event which can be converted into a lesson for preventing such an episode in the future.

This same attitude of justifiable optimism can be applied to the other special problems which some patients face, such as the disturbances of the nervous system, the tendency to blood-vessel complications, and the localized reactions at the site of insulin injection which produce swelling and/or loss of the tissues under the skin.

1.   Nervous system problems in the diabetic (neuritis and neuropathy)

It has long been realized that it is not enough to prevent acidosis and coma to assure the complete health of the patient. Diabetes must be regulated as completely as possible. If this goal is not achieved, the patient may develop signs and symptoms of nervous-system disorder. These might consist of peculiar sensations in the hands and feet and changed bowel habits manifested as constipation or diarrhea with the latter occurring more often at night, unusual patterns of sweating, weakness or paralysis of certain muscles such as those of the bladder or eye, decreased sexual function, and even strange emotional and mental behavior. The exact mechanism of these disorders is not yet clearly understood, but their relationship to poor control of diabetes appears likely. It is known, however, that high blood-sugar levels raise the glucose within nerves. There it is converted to sorbitol and in turn to fructose. This is called the polyol pathway. When the level of glucose in nerves is greatly elevated, the slow conversion of sorbitol to fructose results in an accumulation of sorbitol. The high sorbitol levels result in damage to the nerve sheaths and to the nerves themselves. If the nerve fiber dies, and repair by the body is possible, it takes about a year for a new nerve to develop.

When the doctor treats this problem, he relies not only on every detail of the history of such developments but also upon the confirmatory findings present during physical examination. He may test the sensation of touch, the ability to distinguish between heat and cold, the perception of the vibrations of a tuning fork, the sweating response, the functions of the nerves of the head, the reflexes obtained by striking the ankles, knees, etc. with a rubber hammer, and even the ability of the blood vessels to adapt to changes in the position of the body. Relying on the patient's own statements and on repeated examinations of the same type, the physician can readily evaluate the status of the patient. Treatment is based on as precise control of the diabetes as possible and includes a trial of certain vitamins and other medications which have proved helpful in other cases of the same type. This may necessitate a variety of treatments before relief is obtained. In a very small percentage of patients, the nervous-system problems may first appear after the diabetes has been brought under control. This is merely a delayed response to the poor control present previously, like the bruise of an auto tire which later results in a flat or a blowout, and does not alter the fundamental problem nor its treatment.

2. The eyes of the diabetic person

Incomplete regulation of diabetes with high blood-sugar levels, ketone bodies, and dehydration changes the shape and surface of the lenses of the eye. This disturbs the acuity of vision and makes the fitting of eyeglasses difficult. This is why the eye doctor waits until the diabetes is stable and the eye tests yield consistent results before prescribing the glasses. These are minor nuisances at most.

Except for such temporary changes in the lenses, the eyes of most persons (99 per cent and more) with diabetes retain normal vision throughout their entire life. It is a fact, of course, that whether or not diabetes is present, the lenses of the eye become less flexible and less transparent as the years pass and the senior citizen years set in. It is also true that glaucoma, with increase in eyeball pressure, develops more often in the older person. Moreover, hardening of the arteries, including those of the eyes, accompanies aging. All these changes occur whether or not diabetes is present, and some of them may occur earlier in the person with diabetes. The problem then is not the prevention of these changes, since they are an inevitable accompaniment of living long enough to get old or older whether or not diabetes is present. Rather, the problem is how to delay these changes when diabetes is present.

It is reasonable to hope, but certainly not proved, that avoidance of very high blood sugars may or will help the prevention of cataracts in children and young adults.

It is a fact that periodic checks on eyeball tension by your doctor will identify early increases in pressure which can be permanently controlled by eye drops.

It is highly probable that control of the diabetes by diet, anti-diabetic agents or insulin, and, if need be, administration of certain drugs will keep blood and plasma fats (cholesterol and triglycerides) within the normal range and slow down hardening of the arteries of the eyes.

There remain, however, certain other changes which can or do develop in the eyes of the diabetic that are surely related to the duration of the diabetes and, to an undefined degree, are related to success or failure in maintaining ideal control of the diabetes.

Most of the eye changes which appear in relation to the duration of the diabetes represent no problem as far as vision is concerned. They are minor and insignificant alterations in the size of the veins, insignificant alterations in the channeling of the blood from the arteries to the veins, tiny bulges in these new channels, and insignificant deposits of fat. Some of these changes may appear at the end of the first decade of diabetes, and they are almost invariably present after twenty-five years. These are no more important than freckles. The best proof of this lies in the fact that almost everybody with diabetes of long standing has them to one or another degree, but these usually do not affect the acuity of vision.

Now it is true that a small number of persons with diabetes do develop changes in the eye which do threaten vision. These changes are quite different from all those described above. They consist of new growths of blood vessels, unexpected rupture of these blood vessels with leakage of blood, and formation of a kind of scar tissue. These changes may require special treatment.

Why do some persons (surely less than 1 per cent of all those with diabetes) develop these changes, while others do not? Time again is an element, but not the sole element.

These changes do not appear unless diabetes has been present for a long time, but not all who have had diabetes for a long time develop them. Some believe that time and less than perfect control of diabetes predispose to these changes which threaten vision. This is a very reasonable point of view, since it is often true that the diabetes of such persons is of long duration, that its course has been stormy, and that control has often been less than ideal. However, in fairness to the individual person and in keeping with the fact, it is also true that (1) such severe changes may develop in mild and apparently perfectly controlled diabetes and (2) that none may be seen after many years of inadequate attention to the diabetes. However, prudence dictates that every attempt be made to regulate the diabetes perfectly, since there are examples that support the idea that inadequate control of diabetes may lead to eye problems.

What practical measures can then be taken to avoid these vision-threatening changes? There are these:

1. Postponement of onset of diabetes as long as possible;

2. Early diagnosis and treatment of diabetes;

3. Ideal treatment of diabetes with diet, pills, or insulin with adequate control of urine and blood sugar;

4. Regular visits to your physician and to the eye specialist;

5. Early recognition of vision-threatening changes

Now, it is true that a small number of persons with diabetes do develop changes in the eye which do threaten vision. They consist of new growths of blood vessels, unexpected rupture of these blood vessels with leakage of blood, and formation of a kind of scar tissue. These changes represent "vision threatening retinopathy." These require special treatment, including Laser beam therapy and, in some patients, eye surgery.

Why do some persons (less than 1% of all those with diabetes) develop these changes and others do not? Time again is an element, but not the sole element. These changes do not appear unless diabetes has been present for a long time, but not all who have had diabetes for a long time develop them. Most doctors believe that time and less than perfect control of diabetes predispose to these changes which threaten vision.

3.   The kidneys in diabetes

In more than 99 per cent of persons with diabetes the kidneys remain completely functional and entirely adequate for the full Biblical three score and ten years, and, if need be, for decades longer. In addition to performing all the functions that the kidneys ordinarily perform, these organs take on and complete the special tasks posed to them by diabetes. Indeed, they may even acquire special abilities which help them cope with problems stemming from diabetes.

There is some evidence in support of and some against the view that the kidneys of the diabetic person may show another more or less characteristic change when the diabetes appears and even before it appears. The actual time of appearance of this change is less important than the fact that early in the course of diabetes, perhaps several years or less, the change does develop. Ultimately the change is present in all diabetic persons. This change consists of a thickening of the basement membrane of the kidneys. In this limited degree the thickening of the basement membrane has no harmful effect on the ability of the kidneys to perform their work. This is true even when protein appears in the urine as a sign of this change.

It is a fact, however, that in some individuals, perhaps because the diabetes has not been adequately controlled, the kidneys can fail. This used to be a critical unsolved problem but this is no longer true. Now chronic and irreversible kidney failure or uremia in diabetes can be solved as readily as it has been solved in so many non-diabetic patients, *i.e.* by a kidney transplant. Until recently such kidney transplants were only rarely available to the diabetic patient because early attempts were only partially successful. Now it is proved that careful selection of the donor kidney and appropriate supportive measures markedly improve the success rate. Once the transplant has begun to function adequately, the uremia disappears in the course of a return to normal kidney function. Also, in many instances, the prohibitive hospitalization and other costs of such transplants have been largely solved. Such persons are now eligible for Social Security, Medicare and related financial support to supplement in very important measure their personal and insurance resources. The Kidney Foundation, listed in your metropolitan telephone directory, is very knowledgeable in identifying the institutions and the sources of financial and other aid available in such emergencies.

However, as alluded earlier, there are some tasks that are better performed by the kidneys of a diabetic person. Thus, it has been established that early in diabetes the kidneys do a better than normal job in forming the fluid which represents the first stages of urine.

Also, the kidney of the diabetic person develops an above-average ability to reabsorb sugar from this fluid.

4. Large blood-vessel problems in the patient with diabetes ⤸

All of the inhabitants of the United States, with or without diabetes, face a special blood vessel hazard. Ailments of the arteries of the heart, kidneys and brain are the chief causes of illness in our nation, surpassing even the cancer problem in magnitude. The search for the cause of these ailments is being carried on by far the largest number of scientists engrossed in any medical problem today. As readers of the daily newspaper, as family members, as neighbors and as contributors to the good work of our hospitals and organizations such as the American Heart Association, we are constantly made aware of this hazard to our health and to the health of our loved ones. The vital statistics suggest, though this is not certain, that perhaps never in the history of mankind has any people been beset with this problem to a similar degree.

Hardening of the large arteries, also called atherosclerosis, arteriosclerosis, or macroangiopathy occurs somewhat earlier in the diabetic than in the non-diabetic and may be more extensive. Such large vessel lesions in the heart, brain, feet and elsewhere predispose to heart attacks (myocardial infarcts), strokes, and gangrene.

Prevention includes control of the diabetes by diet, oral anti-diabetic pills or insulin and maintenance of ideal cholesterol and triglyceride levels, i.e. fats, in the plasma.

High total serum cholesterol and total triglyceride levels increase the risk of heart attacks, strokes, etc. as circulating molecules which contain these fats are deposited in the inner walls of the arteries and interfere with blood flow.

Control of the blood sugar, an ideal body weight, careful attention to the amount and kind of fat in the diet (high in unsaturated and low in saturated fat), and normal levels of cholesterol and triglycerides protect against the macroangiopathy.

New evidence indicates that in the population as a whole a high level of HDL-cholesterol (High Density Lipoprotein Cholesterol) is also protective because it means that cholesterol is being transported out of the walls of the blood vessels. This tells us that large blood vessel problems in the diabetic are not only preventable but also, if treated early enough, reversible.

In addition, it may be that a usual kind of heart problem can develop in a diabetic whose coronary arteries are open and whose blood pressure and heart valves are normal. In the small number of patients reported to date the heart muscle enlarges and its pumping efficiency fails. This is a form of idiopathic cardiomyopathy.

The patients with diabetes and idiopathic cardiomyopathy usually have also had small blood vessel circulation problems (microangiopathy) in the kidneys with protein in the urine. This suggests that similar microangiopathy in the heart muscle could be responsible for the heart enlargement and heart failure. Measurements of the efficiency of the left heart chamber and ultrasound studies of the movements of heart muscle and valves also suggest that abnormalities occur only in diabetic patients with microangiopathy and are not evident in those without microangiopathy.

Idiopathic cardiomyopathy is still incompletely understood and can develop in the absence of diabetes. Its apparent close relationship to diabetes does provide, however, another reason for close supervision and control of the blood sugar and any chemical, i.e. metabolic abnormalities.

5. The minor problem of localized reactions to insulin

Rarely, insulin may produce hives and reddening and irritation of the skin surface. This is a sensitivity to the tiny amounts of protein other than insulin left during the manufacture of the hormone, protein such as globin or protamine combined to insulin, or to the insulin itself. This may be accompanied by some difficulty in regulating the diabetes, but the entire problem can usually be avoided by changing to Lente insulin derived from hog rather than beef pancreas. The physician may also prescribe drugs such as the antihistamines or the cortisone-type steroids to control the allergic reactions or avoid them entirely in the non-insulin-dependent person by transferring them to the oral anti-diabetic agents.

There are two other types of localized reaction to insulin which appear as a swelling at the injection site or as a loss of the fatty tissue lying just under the skin. These are of minor importance. Their existence has been recognized ever since insulin became available. The changes appear in some children, both boys and girls, and less often in adults and then almost always in women. Though in certain patients such local tissue changes may interfere with the regulation of diabetes, this is rare. From the viewpoint of prevention it is usually recommended that in susceptible persons the sites of insulin injection be rotated to minimize the swelling and the subsequent loss of fat in any one area. This may, however, increase the number of areas involved and hence in some patients it might be better to continue to inject the insulin into the same area. Placing the insulin injection deep into the muscle is helpful. If these precautions fail to work, there is no need for concern. People are whole persons and personalities and it is only the most vain of us who would think that a slight swelling or irregularity of an arm or leg will make a real difference in our lives or in our relationships with others.

6. Insulin resistance

Rarely, some patients may develop marked resistance to insulin, requiring thousands of units daily. Such patients however still respond with a lowering of the blood sugar if enough insulin is given.

Treatment includes changing to Lente insulin of hog origin, trial of oral anti-diabetic agents if the diabetes responds to these drugs, and administration of antihistaminics and cortisone-type steroids.

12 : INFECTIONS AND SURGERY IN DIABETES

In the period before sulfa drugs and antibiotics it was not infrequent to see a patient develop a series of skin infections or "boils" which required poulticing and drainage. Though it is proper for the physician and the patient to keep the possible relationship of such infections to diabetes in mind, these problems are, of course, by no means confined to those with diabetes.

1. Are patients with diabetes more liable to infections?

As a matter of fact we are not at all sure that, save for the possible exceptions discussed below, diabetes by itself does predispose to such infection. There never were any adequate statistics gathered on this point in the days before treatment of infections with sulfa drugs and penicillin and related agents became available, and there are many ways in which a

134

false impression might have been created. Supposing, for example, that diabetics always reported such infections to their doctor whereas nondiabetics did not. Or, as is likely, let us assume that diabetics brought their skin infection problems to the few doctors specializing in diabetes while nondiabetics were scattered among the practices of many physicians. Either of those factors—and many others could be mentioned—would serve to bolster an erroneous notion that well-regulated patients as a whole are especially prone to skin infections.

Females with diabetes who are poorly regulated, on the other hand, may develop localized infections of the external genitals. These begin as an irritation produced by the passage of large amounts of urine which contains sugar. Hair-follicle infections, boils or fungus infections may develop in such irritated skin. It should be emphasized, however, that this is a local problem in female patients and not a systemic effect of diabetes, resulting for example from a high level of sugar in the blood. It does not occur in males with equally uncontrolled diabetes, nor is the localized irritation in the female accompanied by infections in distant parts of the body. Such localized infections may predispose, however, to infections of the urinary passages, i.e., of the bladder, kidneys and related passages, and therefore should always receive prompt and adequate treatment.

There is another hazard which occurs more often in diabetes but is not peculiar to this condition: this is the possibility of starting a local infection or abscess by means of an improperly sterilized needle. This can happen to anyone who is subjected to frequent injections, and is not confined to those with diabetes.

2.   Prevention and treatment of infections in diabetes

The prevention and treatment of skin infections in anyone, with or without diabetes, involves first cleanliness and good personal hygiene. Prompt and proper treatment of minor scratches and of skin injuries is necessary. If irritation of the external genitals develops in a female patient, this is a sign that the diabetes is uncontrolled. This should be corrected, but recovery can be hastened by proper local hygiene, using tap-water lavage after each passage of urine and applying a salve selected by the doctor for its specific ability to control the bacterial and the fungus infections. Abscesses at injection sites can be avoided by the use of proper sterile techniques in handling the needle, syringe, insulin, etc. (see Chapter 5). When such abscesses appear or the patient develops a serious bacterial infection of any type, the physician will advise the use of penicillin or a related drug. Should the infection prove resistant to treatment it is possible to determine in the laboratory which of the many antibacterial agents available today is most suitable in a particular infection.

Having decided that, save for the exceptions cited, neither diabetes itself nor high blood sugar levels in the patient causes infections, it is wise to emphasize again that infections can and do upset the regulation and control of diabetes. In Chapter 7 it has been pointed out that this can be readily corrected by increasing the total dosage and by shifting, under the guidance of the physician, to short-acting insulin. Such a shift permits prompt readjustments in accordance with the results of urine and blood sugar tests.

It is reasonable to ask whether such disruption of diabetes control by infections in turn interferes with the healing of infections. The answer is Yes if the loss of control results in large enough deficits of water, minerals, vitamins, proteins and other essential body constituents. On the other hand it appears unlikely that a simple rise in blood sugar without such deficits interferes with the healing of a superficial abscess, though it will obviously hinder the clearing of an inflammation of the external genitals in the female or of the urinary passages.

However, the occurrence of "shin spots" or tiny pigmented scars on the lower legs suggests that, for unknown reasons, the healing of tiny skin injuries may take a longer time in some persons with diabetes.

3. Surgery in diabetes

Any of the minor or major surgical events such as a simple wound or the need for the surgical removal of an acute appendicitis which may befall the nondiabetic can also occur in a diabetic. Today, whether these prove catastrophic or not usually depends on their intensity and severity, rather than upon the presence or absence of diabetes. It was not always so: there was a time when they represented special hazards to the diabetic. These have been greatly reduced by the advent of effective means of diabetic therapy and the development of better clinical judgment, safer anesthesia, more effective surgical techniques, rational programs of blood and fluid replacement, the discovery of agents such as heparin which in case of need can prolong the clotting of blood, and the development of sulfa drugs and antibiotics such as penicillin for the control of infections.

Any problems or risks still encountered by the diabetic who develops an infection or requires surgery are directly attributable to three factors which are peculiar to, or occur more often in, the diabetic. These consist of the possibility of inadequate diabetic regulation, the tendency to a higher incidence of vascular problems, and the chance of derangements of nervous-system function, particularly the increase or loss of the sensation of pain in a chronically irritated, inflamed or infected area.

A. MINOR OR MAJOR PROBLEMS

Minor surgery in the diabetic such as removal of skin tumors, repair of simple injuries, and extraction of teeth presents no special problem. It does require, or course, proper preparation. This may include shifting to rapid-acting insulin and provision of water and of food substitutes by vein (glucose solutions) for the period of anesthesia and unconsciousness when the patient cannot and should not drink or eat. If this is not done, the patient who tries to eat or drink may vomit as a result of the anesthesia, drugs, or the surgery itself, and then insulin shock might occur. The usual practice is to stop all intake of food and fluids by mouth from supper until the next morning. At that time part of the insulin dosage is given with an injection of glucose in water. The rest of the insulin and glucose in water is then given after the operation or even during it, if it is prolonged. Frequently the blood-sugar level is measured prior to, during, or after the trip to the operating room as a guide to the treatment. Once the patient is conscious and can take and retain fluids, the injections of glucose solution are replaced by tea, sweetened drinks, fruit juices, milk, etc., which supply calories approximately equal to the amounts present in the patient's usual diet.

Exactly the same preparations are made for major surgery such as delivery of a normal pregnancy by caesarean section, removal of a gall bladder, setting of a fracture, etc. If the operation lasts for a number of hours, more than one measurement of the blood sugar may be made. Also the recovery and healing period may take longer.

B. SPECIAL PROBLEMS IN THE SURGERY OF DIABETICS

In both the so-called minor and the real major surgical problems, loss of diabetic control will interfere with healing as it does in the case of infections. The resultant losses of water and the other important body constituents retard the normal process of repair. Hence non-emergency surgery is always postponed until regulation is satisfactory and this may also have to be done in the emergency procedures. This caution is well-advised.

Those with or without diabetes who have developed hardening of the arteries in the areas where the operation is to be performed obviously require special attention. This is also necessary when the blood vessels of distant organs such as the kidney have been involved. The surgeon selects the anesthetic with care. In local anesthesia, for example, pain-deadening drugs which cause spasm of the blood vessels are avoided. Agents such as heparin which slow down the natural tendency of blood to clot may be given. If the area cannot be made surgically clean before or during the operation, penicillin or related drugs are used.

A few patients with or without vascular disease of the legs may develop clots in the smaller blood vessels following minor injury or with slight infections. These interfere with the circulation and cause the tissues to turn dark. This has been called gangrene. It used to be a far more frequent and often a major problem before the days of penicillin and similar drugs, the availability of agents which control blood clotting, and the development of the new surgical techniques which can increase the circulation to the involved area. Many of these heal, however, with just good medical treatment. These significant improvements in the treatment of such foot problems by no means eliminate the need for good foot hygiene in diabetes. This begins with comfortable clean socks, proper-fitting shoes, careful trimming of toenails to prevent ingrowth and infection, avoiding the cutting of corns and calluses, the prevention of injury by using safety shoes, and prompt medical attention to the slightest injury or infection.

Patients whose sensations in the feet are not normal should be especially careful because injury, infection or ulcers can develop without pain. The absence of this warning signal allays the concern of the patient and defers the necessary visit to the doctor. This should never be allowed to happen.

13 : SOCIAL ASPECTS OF DIABETES

To anticipate some of the problems which may arise in living with diabetes mellitus and to indicate how they can affect the family and friends, certain social aspects of diabetes, behavior on "dates," problems in traveling, and the question of alcoholic beverages are discussed in this chapter.

1. The responsibility of the hostess and the lady of the house

Both the hostess and the housewife can do much to simplify the provision of food for a guest with diabetes if a few common-sense principles are kept in mind.

A. THE HOSTESS

If you invite a friend with diabetes to dine at your home or, more informally, to take potluck with the family, you can do much to help your guest abide by his diet without imposing a hardship on your family. This does not mean you

141

have to provide a set of diabetic scales or go out and purchase foods packed without added sugar. There are only several rules of thumb which ought to be observed. These can best be presented by discussing the various courses of a meal.

1. *Soups and appetizers:* Your guest can have clear bouillon, consomme or broth without restriction, whereas creamed or other more substantial soups will contain a variable amount of carbohydrate, fat and protein. The guest who is following a diet will be faced with two major problems if he accepts the latter: first, there is no way in which the actual amount of the various foodstuffs in a cup or plate of such soup can be estimated; second, if he does know the exact composition (and this information is hard to come by because everybody makes soup his own way, or if it is Mr. Campbell's or Mr. Heinz's product to begin with, it is often "doctored" by adding milk, butter, etc.), these food items and calories will have to be subtracted from the main portion of this or some other meal.

The matter of calculating the food values of shrimp cocktail, oysters on the half-shell, or chopped liver is simple, but again it will limit the intake during the remainder of the meal. If the appetizer is grapefruit, it complicates, as we shall see, the problem of supplying a dessert. Hence the most acceptable substitute for clear soups is one of the fruit or vegetable juices.

2. *The entree:* Casserole dishes are largely taboo, because of the difficulty in knowing precisely what the contents are. This does not mean that the guest can't have them at home where the food is weighed or estimated before the particular delicacy is prepared. With this main restriction the guest can partake of any of the standard meat, poultry or fish dishes,

though ham should not be glazed with pineapple juice nor fish covered with butter sauce. Dressings prepared with bread, meat, chestnuts, oysters, etc., present the same problem as casseroles, though of course here the guest has the option of passing them by. The hostess need not worry herself about the size of the portion because an excess can be left uneaten and seconds are usually available. The accompanying vegetables can be any of the usual family favorites, seasoned to taste but not served creamed nor with hollandaise or other sauces. These can, of couse, be available on the table for those who are not faced with diabetic or caloric restrictions. Obviously, candied sweet potatoes or yams are forbidden.

3. *Relishes, salads, and related items:* Celery, lettuce, tomatoes, cucumbers or pickles can usually be taken freely by your guest and this is true of all the leafy or other simple salads. The dressing should be served separately so that it may be applied as desired. Fruit and cottage-cheese salads, those with nuts, prunes, beets, or gelatin may or may not present a problem and if possible are best eliminated on this one occasion.

4. *Desserts:* Many diabetics can have ordinary ice cream if this is estimated in the total food intake. Special diabetic ice cream or sherbet prepared with saccharine is available but it usually has to be sought out and it may or may not be relished by the other guests. Cakes, eclairs, cookies, pies and puddings should not be offered, though the family may often prepare them as a low-carbohydrate item at home. The easiest solution is fresh fruit because this is the guest's usual dessert and from the point of view of body-weight control other members of the family would do well to confine themselves to this dessert also.

5. *Breakfast and lunch:* If the guest remains overnight or for the week end, the preparation of breakfast and lunch is no problem if these same principles are kept in mind. The custom of the nighttime raid on the refrigerator presents no challenge to the properly indoctrinated guest.

6. *Between-meal snacks:* If the guest is going to stay for several hours or days or if, as happens in the best regulated households, meals are delayed, it is both polite and essential to make milk, fruit juice and simple crackers available as before-meal, between-meal, or bedtime snacks.

If the family customs are casual, with meals on a catch-as-catch-can basis, the cautious guest will prefer to have his lunch or dinner at home or elsewhere before making his social visit. The proper hostess will accept this as a medical necessity and not as a reflection on her culinary art.

If worse comes to worst, and all of the considerate behavior just outlined does not work out, the lady of the house should not feel guilty: in the final analysis it is the guest who is responsible for his own well-being and in our experience even the children are ready to assume this at a remarkably early age. Nor should the hostess be chagrined if the guest ignores her preparations entirely. He may be on a free or normal diet as prescribed by his physician.

B. THE HOUSEWIFE

Initially, of course, a scale and dietetic foods may be required in preparing food for the patient. In many instances this is a temporary phase until she and the patient learn to use household measures or to estimate the food, or until the physician suggests sharing of the food served at the family table. In any case it is good psychology not to have a double standard of eating in the household, with candy and cake for some and not for others.

2. Proper "date" behavior

This does not, of course, refer to whether it is proper to kiss the boy friend on the first night out. It might be well however, for those with diabetes not to date others with diabetes, since if marriage results the two diabetics are very likely to have children with diabetes. Here, however, we are getting way ahead of our story which started out, after all, as a discussion of the social amenities. Back then to the problem of how to be at the same time an unobtrusive patient and socially acceptable, without compromising the principles of proper diabetic living.

First there ought to be no concern about keeping secret or disclosing the fact that you have diabetes. This information should be allowed to come out naturally as it often will if the patient is totally at ease about the matter. Such an attitude will avoid the necessity of discussing the subject with casual acquaintances and there will be no pressure about informing more intimate friends.

The problem of going out to dinner with a "date" can be readily resolved by selecting appropriate items from the menu in accordance with the patient's own knowledge of the diet. The new and inexperienced patient will find some useful general principles in the preceding section which provides advice to a hostess on how to entertain a diabetic guest.

The end-of-the-evening snack should present no difficulties. As a matter of fact, patients who are on intermediate insulin, or mixtures which have the same action—and these make up the bulk of the younger group—usually take a substantial feeding at night, say 25 grams of carbohydrate, in addition to fat and protein, consisting of a sandwich and a drink. Hence a hamburger and a glass of milk will fill the bill both socially and medically. In the case of patients not on insulin only a simple rearrangement of the evening meal will provide food for the late-evening snack.

Obviously, common sense must always prevail if shocking is to be avoided. When the evening's activity is to consist of strenuous skating or bowling, additional amounts of food can and should be taken. Also, the emergency ration of carbohydrate to offset unexpected low blood sugars must be at hand.

3. The traveling patient

The availability of urine sugar tests which require no external heat such as Tes-Tape®, Chemstrip® or Clinitest® (see Appendix) and of sterile disposable syringes and needles allows the patient to travel freely for days by car, train, or plane. The insulin supply can be kept chilled in the refrigerator of the hotel or motel and on the train or plane. In between times, it should be carried in an insulated bag of the type supplied for ice cream. If very hot weather is expected, a packet of dry ice available in many fountains or dairy stores will serve as well. With regard to meals, it is wise to take along substitute nonperishable food if the train has no diner or the plane fails to deliver the meal (or the passenger!) on time as promised in the schedule. As indicated earlier, a readily accessible identification bracelet or care indicating that the wearer has diabetes is good insurance in case of injury or unexpected emergency.

4. The problem of alcoholic beverages

Nowadays hospitality often includes cocktails or other alcoholic beverages. Alcohol is consumed in the body as if it were a fat and hence by itself does not increase the insulin requirement. The difficulty insofar as the patient is concerned is that the alcohol, the fruit and the sugar in such a drink must be counted as calories which must be subtracted from the assigned diet. Then there is the problem of the loss of judgment which everyone except perhaps the drinker himself admits occurs with drinking. This can cause errors and mistakes in regulating the diabetes. Finally, if an insulin shock or other catastrophe should occur, it is very logical for any good Samaritan to conclude from the odor on the breath that the person is intoxicated and just needs to sleep it off. Probably it is best for the patient to avoid alcohol altogether but in any case great care and judgment should be exercised in its use. Your friends will accept and respect your attitude when the reasons for avoiding alcohol are made apparent.

14: DIABETES IN CHILDREN

Diabetes of children is often called Juvenile Onset Diabetes (JOD). It occurs in 1.3 out of each 1000 children of school age. Most often this is insulin deficient and hence is called Juvenile Insulin Dependent Diabetes (JIDD). However, some children can develop mild diabetes of the adult-onset or maturity onset type. It is then called Maturity Onset Diabetes of Youth (MODY) or Maturity Onset Hyperglycemia of Youth (MOHY).

Though most adults develop Adult-Onset or Maturity Onset Diabetics (AOD or MOD), some can develop the insulin dependent type.

1. Which child is especially apt to develop diabetes?

Among adults, overweight predisposes to the development of diabetes. There is no such relationship apparent in children: diabetes occurs with equal frequency among those who are underweight, or normal weight, or overweight.

2. Do infections cause diabetes in children?

Physicians have long known that mumps infection may damage the pancreas in man and produce diabetes. Also, in animals, mixing certain viruses can in the test tube kill the insulin-producing cells of the pancreas. In recent years it has been established that virus infections in mice can induce diabetes. This is more apt to happen if the mice have an increased tendency to spontaneous diabetes as a result of in-breeding.

Evidence that virus infections such as mumps, German measles, Coxsackie B virus, etc. precede the appearance of childhood diabetes is now being accumulated. Thus, epidemics of mumps may be followed by an increased number of new cases of diabetes. This is also true of isolated cases of mild measles or of Coxsackie B infections.

Much progress has been made in identifying those children in whom there is a greater risk that a virus infection will be followed by diabetes. Thus, on Chromosome #6 there are 4 sites or loci whose antigens (Human Leucocyte Antigens or HLA) have been inherited in pairs from 1 parent or the other. Hence, a person may have inherited, for example, B6 and C15 from one parent and A7 and D11 from the other. The numbers cited are only a few of the many possible combinations and only in identical twins would the antigens be the same.

Study of these 4 loci in children with insulin dependent diabetes (JIDD) has revealed that in the United States certain pairs of antigens, B8 and Bw15, for example, occur more often than they do in nondiabetics and that others are less frequent. This suggests that chromosomes do play a role in this type of diabetes and that a B8-Bw15 combination, or other combinations of A, B, C and D antigens in other parts of the world or in different ethnic groups predispose to damage by viruses or by other factors.

3. Diabetes among relatives of children with diabetes

Diabetes mellitus is not a single genetic trait and heredity, when present, is polygenic and multifactorial.

In the case of twins the age at onset of diabetes in one of them determines what happens to the other. Thus, when diabetes appears in one of the twins before the age of 40 the other may or may not develop diabetes, i.e. 50% are concordant and 50% are discordant. If, however, the diabetes appears after the age of 40, the concordant frequency is 90%.

Juvenile Insulin Dependent Diabetes (JIDD) and Maturity Onset Diabetes of Youth (MODY) or Maturity Onset Hyperglycemia of Youth (MOHY) differ in intensity. Thus, MODY or MOHY is mild diabetes which usually does not require insulin treatment because the patient still secretes insulin. It does not become more severe or progress to JIDD. Acidosis does not occur. In JIDD on the other hand there is a critical shortage of insulin, the diabetes is severe and acidosis occurs if insulin is not injected.

The family histories in MODY or MOHY or JIDD also indicate that they are two separate disorders because these two types of diabetes in children or young adults have different genetic patterns. Thus, in MODY or MOHY there is a history of diabetes in three generations of the family in about 45% of the patients, one or the other parent is diabetic in 85% instances, and 55% of the patients have a brother or sister with either obvious diabetes or high blood sugar levels. The corresponding frequencies in JIDD are only about 6%, 10%, and 10%. These statistics clearly establish that the hereditary aspects are quite different in MODY and

MOHY and JIDD.

Hence, in current thinking JIDD occurs in persons who inherit weak pancreatic islets, abnormal immune responses, or other traits which increase significantly the risk of diabetes, probably, as indicated, as a result of islet damage.

4. At what age does childhood diabetes appear?

In a group of some 600 children treated to date in our clinic, the average age at onset was eight years in girls as well as in boys (figure 13). In contrast to adult women who tend

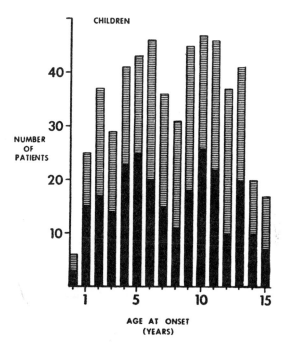

DIABETES IN CHILDREN: AGE AT ONSET.

In children, the average age at onset of diabetes is 8 years. However there is indication in the above figure that the 5-year old and the 10-year old girls may be especially susceptible (note the peaks at those two periods). (Figure 13) Horizontal markings identify boys.

to develop diabetes more often than men, female infants and children of all ages are no more susceptible than the males. In girls, however, there may be—and this is not certain—a greater tendency for diabetes to first appear at the ages of five and ten. We have also taken care of infants and young children whose diabetes began between the ages of one and three years of age or even earlier. This group makes up about 10 per cent of our total population of juvenile patients. In other clinics, as in the one conducted by Dr. George Guest at Cincinnati, diabetes has been diagnosed within the first few hours of life.

5. What are the first signs of diabetes in childhood?

Diabetes is ushered in during childhood with many of the same signs that can appear in adults except that they are apt to be more frequent and more marked. As an example, increased passage of urine, thirst, weight loss and weakness, which may be totally absent in many adult patients, are present individually or in combination in about 90 per cent of the affected children. Other clues such as irritable behavior or return of bed wetting may also appear. The relative frequency of these and other manifestations is shown in figure 14. Since symptoms do occur more often in children and arouse the concern of parents and the doctor, it is not surprising to find that diabetes is usually diagnosed more promptly in children than in adults. About one-half of our diagnosed children were identified within a month or less of the probable onset of the diabetes, but delays were present in others because in the group as a whole three months passed on the average before the cause of the symptoms was ferreted out. This delay is always undesirable but especially so in the

ONSET SYMPTOMS
TOTAL NUMBER OF PATIENTS-513

Symptom	Percent
← Urination	78
← Thirst	75
Weight Loss	57
Tired	48
← Appetite	44
Night Urination	39
Urine Exam	31
Infections	28
Irritability	20
Acidosis-Coma	18
Vomiting	15
Abdominal Pain	13
Colds	13
Bed Wetting	13
Over-Breathing	8

SYMPTOMS IN CHILDREN AT ONSET OF DIABETES. (Figure 14)

In these 513 children with diabetes increased urination and increased thirst were the most common symptoms. (Modified from the author's text, Diabetes Mellitus with Emphasis on Children and Young Adults, *with permission of the publishers, Williams and Wilkins, Baltimore, Md.)*

case of children because it may bring on acidosis and coma. It is not that everyone concerned does not try to find the cause of childhood complaints, but that there may be confusing factors present. It is very easy to be led into thinking that Johnny's illness is the same as his playmate's who has just finished having "flu." The winter with its many colds and respiratory infections is a bad time for many children living in northern climates and it is the time of the year when diabetes is often discovered. However, it may appear during any season.

6. Treatment of diabetes in children

Children with juvenile insulin dependent diabetes (JIDD) need an adequate amount of insulin each day for normal growth and strength. As pointed out earlier, many adults, especially those who are overweight, can be treated by diet alone, but children cannot have their diet markedly restricted if they are to develop normally. As a matter of fact, though diet is always important in the treatment of diabetes in children, it is nowhere near as important as the insulin injections. It has been shown, for example, that children with good eating habits can have the same foods that are served to the rest of the family and do well, provided the insulin dosage is regulated properly. This is not to say that such a program is recommended for all affected children, nor, as a matter of fact, for any of them. This is a matter to be settled by the doctor or the clinic in charge and usually involves careful prescription of the foods eaten in accord with the American Diabetes Association or similar diets. Irrespective of the dietary program used, all of these children also receive insulin. Furthermore, the currently available substitutes for insulin which may be effective when taken by mouth by many adult patients are only rarely useful or used in childhood diabetes.

There is no reason why any child should go hungry. The proper diet will not only meet the growth and energy needs but will satisfy the hunger as well. It includes between-meal and after-play snacks and even provides for the social demands of a party or a "date."

It is very important to enlist the aid of the family and, as soon as age permits, the active participation of the child in the care of the diabetes. Many youngsters learn to run urine tests and to inject their own insulin before they are ten years of age. At about this time or shortly thereafter they are ready to adjust their insulin dosage in accord with the results of urine tests and can compensate for changes in diabetes brought about by illnesses, menstrual periods, emotional upsets, etc. Throughout this early training it is wise to proceed very calmly and unemotionally in developing self-reliance and the proper attitudes and habits.

7. What is the pay-off of proper diabetic care of childhood diabetes?

Parents of any child with a lifetime disorder tend, consciously or unconsciously, to feel guilty. This may lead to undue solicitude for the diabetic child. Such constant concern and an overprotective attitude may suppress the emotional maturation of the child and lead to passive and dependent behavior. On the other hand, the normal process of growing up involves setting oneself up as an independent individual. Undue solicitude can either inhibit this normal process or lead to adolescent rebellion in which the diabetes regimen serves as a family battlefield. This can all be avoided by a calm and trusting attitude on the part of the parents and child that diabetes is compatible with perfectly normal growth, development, and adult life. Statistics from our group of patients and other clinics indicate that with adequate care the treated child can be expected to increase in height and weight at a rate which falls within the normal range, be of normal intelligence, earn good grades in school, develop normally from the point of view of emotions and sex, participate in sports, learn the skills of a trade or profession, marry and have children. All of this lies ahead of the properly guided children and can be achieved despite the fact that in the face of the very best of care occasional acidosis and coma and eye and kidney problems may occur.

15 : PREGNANCY IN DIABETES

From a narrow, but certainly a long-term point of view, we exist in nature as perpetuators of the human species. Since time immemorial the birth of a child has signified another chance for the parents as individuals, for the relatives as a family, for a people as a race, and for man as a human being. The slate has been wiped clean for a fresh start: a new house has been provided for the grand hopes of mankind. Certainly the first child with diabetes, whoever it may have been, who with the help of insulin lived long enough to become a mother or a father represented an unrecorded but none-theless dramatic moment in the history of mankind. A thread of life, hitherto wasted, became available. In this land where all are born with equal rights and with unlimited hopes, what other response can be given to the question, "Should those with diabetes have a family" except "Yes"? And, it is easy to give this answer. The risk to the diagnosed mother is, if anything less than in the population as a whole. This does not mean, of course, that there are no problems nor that common sense based on experience can be ignored. What then are the problems faced in starting a family?

1. The higher rates of pregnancy loss in diabetes

The facts are clear on the point that diabetes runs in families. If two people with diabetes marry (and any marriage counselor can demonstrate that left to their own devices they'd certainly do this because like seeks like except when it seeks opposites!), the probability of begetting a child with diabetes is all the greater. The crux of the problem here lies in the fact, to be elaborated upon later, that the chances of successful pregnancies and living offspring are always less in diabetes. It is not that children of such parents are less desirable but rather that they're harder to come by. For this reason it is unwise for those with diabetes to marry others with diabetes.

Even with a nondiabetic mate a diabetic may encounter problems in starting a family. It has long been recognized that the diagnosed female can be expected to have a higher rate of uncompleted pregnancies and may even have trouble becoming pregnant. If she is successful, there is no point, even at the very time of birth, when anxiety for the welfare of the child can be relaxed. Again the statistics are clear: among such mothers the percentage of miscarriages and deaths of babies before or even after birth is distinctly higher than in those without diabetes. Though with excellent care this risk can be decreased, it still exists.

2. Problems of regulation during pregnancy

Even though it has been emphasized, and it is true, that there is no risk to the mother, this does not mean that pregnancy has no effect on the course of diabetes. There are numerous reports which indicate that in a normal pregnancy

the insulin requirement usually rises, and that the regulation of the diabetes becomes more difficult. Part of this
results from the increased severity in the diabetes brought
about by the hormonal and other changes of pregnancy such
as morning nausea, lessened physical activity, and emotional
factors, and part from the confusion in evaluating the results
of urine tests. More sugar than usual appears in the urine not
only because the diabetes becomes more marked, but also
because blood sugar, i.e. glucose, "spills over" more readily
into the urine; the appearance in the urine of a new sugar
ordinarily present in breast milk (lactose) may also confuse
the picture. The first of these problems is readily met by
increasing the dosage of insulin; the other two will require,
respectively, a temporary revision of the standards of
adequate control and the use of the specific tests for glucose,
such as Tes-Tape®, rather than the time-honored Benedict's
solution or Clinitest®. As pregnancy progresses the diabetes
often becomes milder, returning to its previous state. These
variations require appropriate adjustments in insulin dosage.
Otherwise either acidosis-coma or insulin shock may inter-
rupt the pregnancy. Quite regularly following delivery the
insulin requirement decreases sharply and again shocks must
be avoided. This may be a permanent effect, especially after
the second or subsequent pregnancies.

3. Saving the lives of infants

It is possible to prevent some of the problems faced by the
infants of affected mothers. They tend to be unduly large in
terms of birth weight and yet miniature in terms of
development. If pregnancy is allowed to end by natural
delivery the child may be injured. For this reason it is

recommended that the mother be delivered in the 36th week when the baby is of normal size rather than to await the 40th week. This procedure in addition saves a certain number of infants that die during those crucial last few weeks. Caesarean section is selected for this (and there is no need to worry that there is a real limit to the number of Caesarean operations that can be performed) because this avoids subjecting the child to the bruising and other mild injuries which inevitably accompany even the totally uncomplicated natural birth. It is customary to have a pediatrician stand by at the time of the operation to provide the special attention which may be needed. If all goes well, as many as 90 per cent of the babies may be born and develop normally. If fortune is unkind this number may be reduced to 30 per cent. Science is coming to the aid of these. Thus, measurements of female sex hormones such as estriol in the urine or plasma aid in alerting the physician to impending problems.

4. The prediabetic state

From the above discussion it is clear that the higher-than-normal loss of diabetic pregnancies and the high death rate remain as an unsolved problem of diabetes. At times it has appeared that hormone treatment during pregnancy is the solution, and at times early delivery is just as effective. Certainly the patient should be closely watched and carefully regulated during pregnancy but it looks as if this alone is not enough. Actually, this hazard seems to be related to whatever factor or factors may predispose to diabetes itself. There is considerable evidence that this unfortunate pregnancy record may antedate the appearance of diabetes itself by many years, as "the prediabetic syndrome" and is manifested by frequent miscarriages, the birth of especially large babies, or the death of infants just before or after delivery. During this period there is no diabetes present insofar as we understand the symptoms and signs of this condition. This makes it logical to conclude that, even with the best of medical care and diabetic regulation, there may still be additional unsolved problems in carrying the pregnancy through to a successful conclusion.

There is no comfort to be derived, however, from being a male with diabetes in avoiding these hazards to the infant. Studies in South Africa by Dr. W. P. U. Jackson, questioned in some parts of the world, have suggested that the prediabetic syndrome may also occur in affected males. They become fathers of large babies and their wives give a history of unsuccessful pregnancies similar to those recorded in mothers with diabetes.

5. Facing the facts

After the presentation of facts, insofar as they are now available, what attitude should be taken by the patient, male or female, who contemplates parenthood? In keeping with the general philosophy which we endeavor to inculcate in our patients, the first recommendation is that the facts be faced and the possibility of risks be accepted. Thereafter, all efforts should be concentrated upon following the advice of the very best medical, obstetrical and pediatric care available. Beyond that, the outcome, as with all human affairs, cannot be charted.

16 : LIVING WITH DIABETES:
ATTITUDES AND EXPECTATIONS

1. Attitudes

In being led through the intricacies of diabetes the reader might have quite properly felt overwhelmed at several points. This is a normal reaction to such a mass of new information under any circumstance, and this response is of course accentuated if the reader has a heavy emotional investment in the subject. The latter is naturally true of the patient himself and of his family. However, even though rereading of the complicated portions of this volume—and most people find this necessary—does provide more complete understanding, there still remain the questions of the relative importance and the practical significance of the many aspects of diabetes which have been covered. It is now necessary, therefore, to place the various facets of diabetes as a way of life into their proper perspective.

161

DIABETES: AN EXCUSE, A CLUB, OR AN ASSET?

It is well for all of us, affected or not, to keep in mind the general principle that it is only human to seek an excuse outside ourselves for our personal inadequacies and short-comings. In most instances shirking of home or social responsibilities, poor performance at work, or laziness cannot be blamed on diabetes. It is true that fatigue, irritability and lack of the usual sense of well-being may be manifestations of poor diabetic regulation, arising either from a lack or an excess of insulin. These should be temporary symptoms only and can be expected to disappear—and they do, with proper control. Hence, if such complaints are made by or are noted in a controlled patient, their cause must be sought in other features of his life, i.e. in his attitudes, in her personality, in his drives, in her adjustments to everyday stress, in the demands placed upon him, and in his expectations of himself. The answer may not be easily come by, of course, and may require "cures" for boredom, new goals, reorientation of views, or changes of personal relationships, environment and of employment. Again it should be stressed that these problems, when they arise, are not in any way unique to the patient. They are rather very much a part of everyday living. Recognition of this fact will protect the patient and his family from misunderstandings and, far more important, stimulate a search for remedies to correct personality problems which would otherwise, and erroneously, be blamed on diabetes. In our society it is recognized that such remedial measures may necessitate consultations with teachers, vocational guidance centers, personnel managers, family aid societies, religious advisors, and even psychiatrists.

The latter should not be taken as an implication that there is an invariable personality pattern or, indeed, any defect in the make-up of the diabetic population as a whole. There is no evidence that the patient is fundamentally different from the nondiabetic in this regard. He has all of the strengths, assets, and weaknesses of mankind in general and can be expected to resolve the immediate and long-term problems of existence with as much success as any of us. Regulated diabetes, therefore, cannot be offered nor accepted as an excuse for any of our shortcomings.

Similarly, it is well to be aware of the fact that consciously or unconsciously the patient or his family may use this condition as a club. For example, it might be used as a means of obtaining special consideration or privileges at home or at work. We are not referring, of course, to the dietary and other needs of the patient. These are reasonable. Nor is there anything wrong with avoiding occupations or activities which might prove hazardous to the patient and to people around him should he experience, for example, an insulin shock. This is only common sense. On the other hand, there is no special reason why a patient should be freed of the chores of dishwashing or be allowed special privileges beyond those considered reasonable for any other member of the household or the social community. In meeting these problems as they may arise it is well to keep in mind the harmful effects of temper tantrums and "scenes" not only on the emotional tranquility of the household, the business, or the office, but also their interference with satisfactory and successful diabetic regulation. There are cases on record, for example, of patients who have deliberately brought on an acidosis or coma, or an insulin shock, as a consequence of an emotional scene. In this way they hope to frighten the opposition into compliance or submission. This is obviously an extremely dangerous club to use. In dealing with such problems the ordinary rules of decent behavior should apply. Reasonable people, diabetes notwithstanding, do not make impossible demands of their family or friends, nor do they deny or thwart reasonable requests.

Finally, it is well to keep in mind that diabetes is in many ways an asset. It leads the patient to a more reasonable schedule of living. More attention is paid to regularity of meals, to nourishing foods, to good personal hygiene, to reasonable bedtime hours, to regular health check-ups, and to earlier diagnosis and more prompt treatment of illnesses which can and do occur in any of us.

2. Expectations

What can the patient look forward to? In the preceding chapters many of the problems which may arise in the life of the patient have been discussed. Are they all equally important and what are the chances that any one of them might occur in a particular individual?

First, it should be clear that diabetes by itself is no longer a major hazard to survival. It was not always so, of course. It has already been pointed out earlier, for example, that before insulin became available almost all such children were doomed to an early death in diabetic coma and that this was true in about one-half of the adults. This picture has changed and death in coma has reached the vanishing point in children known to have diabetes.

What are the chances of an acidosis or coma in a diagnosed patient? With proper principles of treatment they are virtually zero in most adults. This is true even though they are exposed to events which could bring on this complication. Good management can and does forestall acidosis and coma and most of our adult patients pass their entire life without experiencing a single episode. In children, however, the need for insulin is so much more definite and changes can occur so rapidly, as they do in many other childhood illnesses, that it may not always be possible to prevent acidosis or coma. Despite this fact it has been our experience that all such children under our care average only one such episode for every five years of known diabetes, and, as indicated earlier, almost always recover promptly.

Though the incidence of coma is less among adults than in children, the average diagnosed adult runs a greater risk. It should be kept in mind, however, that most cases of coma in adults are preventable, and that early treatment and knowledge of other complicating illness greatly reduces this risk. This is, of course, the point in writing and in reading this book. If the principles of proper care are applied in the life of a particular patient, he is no longer exposed to the same hazards, acidosis and coma among them, which are present in the diabetic population as a whole. The latter of necessity includes people who do not even know that they have diabetes or fail to obtain proper attention and care for diagnosed diabetes. It is this group that contributes heavily to the less-than-ideal record.

What are the chances of insulin shock? These are practically zero in patients regulated by diet alone, but occasional reactive hypoglycemia does develop. Also, oral anti-diabetic agents of the sulfonylurea type can produce very low blood sugars. In patients who take insulin, the frequency of shocking depends on irregular habits of diet, physical activity or insulin administration. There are some patients who as a consequence of such irregularities shock every day. This is exactly what our knowledge of insulin action would lead us to expect. These episodes can be prevented by reorganization of the patient's daily schedule and customs. It should be kept in mind, however, that a patient will shock on what may be called an ideal program, if they receive too much insulin. In general it is well to remember that whenever the urines are entirely free of sugar throughout the day and night, insulin shock may be imminent. For this reason it is wise to test for the margin of safety present by occasional decrease in the insulin dosage and allowing some spillage of sugar to occur. All doctors see occasional, but rare, patients in whom the need for insulin has decreased without their knowledge or awareness. A simple test, temporary reduction of the dosage of insulin, will serve to identify such phases and prevent shocking. It is also well to repeat again that, in testing urine, a before-breakfast rather than the overnight specimen should be used as a guide to the adequacy of the dosage of the longer-acting insulin. Insulin shocking should never be ignored. It is a danger signal calling for prompt readjustment of dosage.

Insofar as "neuritis" or related disturbances of nervous function are concerned, these occur only infrequently in diabetics and then almost always in those who are or have been poorly controlled. The well-regulated patient is much less apt to develop this complication.

What are the chances of blood-vessel complications in diabetes? As has already been indicated, all Americans, healthy or not, appear to have high blood pressure and hardening of the arteries of the heart, brain, etc. more often than do populations in certain other parts of the world. It is the chief cause of death in America today with or without diabetes. It is unquestioned that patients run an additional risk of developing these ailments as well as certain diabetes-specific small blood vessel changes in the eyes, kidneys, nerves, and other tissues. Many physicians and clinics feel that adequate regulation of diabetes minimizes this hazard. Hence competent control of diabetes not only keeps the patient free of symptoms of unregulated diabetes and enables him to lead a normal life free of acidosis-coma, insulin shocking and nervous system disorders but also increases the chances of minimizing or eliminating this extra hazard to the blood vessels. Regular visits to the doctor or clinic pay dividends in early treatment of urinary infections, weight control, blood-pressure regulation, eye problems, etc., and further reduce this risk.

The information on patients assembled by the Bureau of Vital Statistics and in various clinics leaves no doubt that year after year the life expectancy of the patient is greater and greater. Taking into account all cases of diabetes, even those that are not diagnosed early or who do not receive adequate care, the life expectancy is within several years of that for the American population as a whole.

Tuberculosis, which used to be a greater hazard to diabetics than to nondiabetics, has decreased almost to the vanishing point in both groups. Also, when all available knowledge is applied, surgical procedures no longer present any special hazards to diabetics. Similarly, the diabetic with an uncomplicated infection such as pneumonia, tonsillitis, etc., responds promptly and adequately to the new wonder drugs.

Perhaps the most striking evidence of the progress that has been made in diabetic regulation has been the ever-expanding list of government and civil-service positions which the diabetic may hold and the fact that diabetics may now purchase life insurance. This is a definite acknowledgment by hardheaded businessmen and government bureaus that diabetics can and do take their proper place in our day-to-day world. We have always known that the well-regulated diabetic was just another human being and that, with proper guidance and effort, he can enjoy a full life.

17 : QUESTIONS AND ANSWERS:
A CHECK LIST FOR PATIENTS

1. *Are you under the care of a doctor or clinic?*

   Though it is true that most of the time diabetes is treated either by the patient or his family, this should always be under the guidance of a physician or clinic. Only in this way can preventive measures be undertaken in time and undue delays in diagnosis and treatment of complications avoided.

2. *Do you understand that body chemistry and chemical reactions are fundamentally the same with or without diabetes?*

   It is important to realize that the body composition and the chemical processes of the patient differ from those of the nondiabetic only in degree and not in kind. For example, the patient can use sugar but the ability in this regard is limited. There are, of course, certain pronounced changes which develop when insulin shortage becomes marked. These involve not only the level of blood sugar but also the concentration, the total amount and the distribution of water and of important chemical constituents such as sodium, potassium, hydrogen ions, etc.

3. *Is it clear that diabetes is never complete or total?*

The patient who has no source of insulin whatsoever, as in the case of someone who has had the pancreas removed surgically for tumor, can still use sugar to a limited degree. In other words, the tissues possess an inherent capacity to carry on the chemical processes necessary for energy, repair, and growth. Insulin increases the rates at which these processes take place but does not initiate them.

4. *Do you know that foods other than starches and sugars are turned to sugar in the body?*

The tissues are capable of producing sugar from protein and, to a limited degree, from the glycerol of fat. This is why in the patient who for one reason or another cannot eat, the blood sugar is still high. Also this accounts for the fact that complete elimination of obvious sugars and starches from the diet may not reduce the blood-sugar levels to normal. This new formation of sugar is a device for providing us with a ready source of energy in periods between eating. In these intervals, stores of protein and of fat are summoned forth for energy purposes. This conversion also explains why in certain unregulated patients there may be much more sugar in the urine than that which is present in the diet.

5. *Do you have increased thirst, increased urination, or is your weight decreasing despite a good appetite?*

These are signs that the diabetes is not completely regulated. As a result the excesses of sugar in the blood spill over into the urine. This increases the volume of urine and decreases the amount of water in the body, resulting in thirst. The weight decrease is a sign that despite ordinary or even increased intake of food, large amounts of calories are being lost in the urine. Glucose lost in this way obviously cannot be used for energy, repair, or growth purposes.

6. *Why not test the blood rather than the urine for sugar?*

As has been indicated elsewhere, the responsibility for day-to-day care of diabetes rests with the patient or with his family. The only practical index of diabetes regulation under such circumstances is urine testing. Blood-sugar tests are expensive, require visits to the doctor, clinic or laboratory, and really do not provide us with all the information necessary for diabetes regulation. They do not tell us, for example, how much sugar is being lost. Also the blood sugar tends to change quickly and hence a sample taken at one moment will not be representative of values present half an hour later. This does not mean that blood-sugar levels are not valuable under certain conditions as, for example, in the diagnosis of diabetes, in differentiating insulin shock and diabetic acidosis, in treating acidosis and coma, and in achieving the close minute-to-minute control needed during operations, or when the urine sugar does not accurately reflect the level of blood sugar..

7. *Why does sugar appear in the urine?*

Each twenty-four hours of the day the units of the kidney filter about 45 gallons of body fluid. In those with or without diabetes and normal blood-sugar levels, all of the sugar in this fluid is reabsorbed by the tubules of the kidney and returned to the body. If the blood sugar becomes elevated above the range characteristic of those with controlled diabetes, then the amount filtered exceeds the capacity of the tubules to reabsorb and sugar appears in the urine.

There are occasional otherwise-healthy individuals who lack the usual ability to reabsorb sugar, and hence spillage occurs at normal blood-sugar levels. This is referred to as "a low threshold" or renal glucosuria. This is not diabetes.

8. *Do you test your urine regularly?*

The patient is in constant need of signposts that the diabetes is adequately regulated. It is true that the presence or absence of symptoms such as thirst, weight loss, excessive urination, provides a rough clue. Regular urine testing, on the other hand, detects trouble before symptoms appear. If circumstances allow, many patients test urine up to four or five times each day. In those that are well controlled it may be possible to reduce the number of tests. In such cases the physician usually still requests a before-breakfast and a before-supper test, but this may be adjusted to meet the patient's individual problem.

9. *Is the sugar in urine always glucose?*

A number of sugars may produce a positive test with Benedict's solution or Clinitest®. This is true of milk sugar present in pregnant women or in nursing mothers, certain sugars found in fruits, and rare types of sugars which appear in the urine as inherited errors of metabolism. Also, nonsugar substances such as penicillin may produce positive tests. Tes-Tape® or Clinistix® readily differentiate glucose from other substances. The identification of other sugars and materials which give positive tests usually requires more extensive laboratory work.

10. *When should urine acetone or ketone-body tests be used?*

When urine acetone or ketone-body tests are positive, they

provide evidence that the body is relying upon fat for energy to a greater extent than usual. They indicate, therefore, that regulation is even less effective than when sugar only is present in the urine. In most cases of diabetes the physician will prescribe the use of acetone tests as an additional guide in treatment.

When acetone is present and the urine sugar is 1+ or zero, the diet may lack sufficient carbohydrate or the patient may be shocking. In either case, the body is once again turning to fat as a fuel.

11. *Can diabetes be controlled by diet alone?*

Diabetes is a spectrum ranging all the way from patients who require strict dietary prescription and large amounts of insulin to those who are adequately controlled by diet alone. The latter almost never occurs in children nor in patients who are thin by nature. In obese patients, on the other hand, body weight reduction will often eliminate the need for insulin.

12. *Are you overweight?*

Any overweight person requires a larger number of calories than a thin person to maintain the body temperature and to perform work. This larger intake of food necessitates a greater supply of insulin. Hence, if the overweight patient does reduce body weight, the needs for calories and insulin also decrease. This reduction may be great enough, and usually is, to allow the patient to be regulated by diet alone. Similarly, it is obvious that weight control, statistically at least, prevents diabetes. However, not all overweight persons develop diabetes nor are all patients overweight at the time the symptoms begin or the diagnosis of diabetes is made.

It is well to point out, however, that our thinking is

changing concerning the role of food intake in overweight patients. It may well be that they possess, in a sense, a more efficient metabolism and therefore tend to put on extra weight without excessive eating, or fail to lose weight despite marked restriction of calories. In a way this is comparable to getting eighteen miles to a gallon of gasoline rather than ten.

13. *Which patients need insulin?*

Despite the generalizations in the preceding two paragraphs on patients as a group, it is usually not possible to predict which individual patient will need insulin and in what quantity. However, patients who have considerable amounts of sugar and acetone surely at that time need insulin. It is highly likely moreover that anyone with a history of diabetic ketoacidosis and coma will require insulin. Also, diabetes incompletely responsive to diet and to oral anti-diabetic agents has to be treated with insulin. The actual dosage is determined by the trial-and-error method with the urine sugar as an index of satisfactory control. At times the blood sugar may be measured to be sure that the urine reflects the blood sugar accurately.

14. *Can insulin be taken by mouth?*

No. However, sulfonylureas (Orinase, Dymelor, Tolinase, and Diabinese) and phenformin (DBI and DBI-TD) taken by mouth can control or aid the control of blood and urine sugar in certain patients. The sulfonylureas act chiefly by increasing the output of insulin from the pancreas and decreasing the secretion of glucagon, a pancreatic hormone that raises blood sugar. Phenformin produces its effect in the main by speeding up the rate at which sugar is used—provided that injected or secreted insulin is present—and by controlling the rate of sugar or absorption from the intestinal tract. Though certain types of diabetes are more responsive than others to oral anti-diabetic agents it is not possible to predict the degree of success in any individual patient. This can only be determined by a trial.

15.*What is U 40, U 80, and U 100 insulin?*

The U refers to units, i.e., each cc (cubic centimeter) or ml (milliliter) contains this number of units of insulin. Hence, U 40 insulin contains 40 units per cc and a 10 cc bottle contains 400 units. U 80 insulin contains 80 units per cc and a 10 cc bottle contains 800 units. It is obvious therefore that U 80 is twice as strong as U 40. The insulin syringe has a graduation for U 40 or U 80 insulin and the proper one should be used in measuring the dosage. It is dangerous to try to use U 80 insulin on a U 40 scale or vice versa because errors are apt to be made. For this reason the medical profession recommends that only U 100 insulin and the new 100 U syringe be used.

16.*How to select an insulin.*

Ultimately this too proves to be a process of trial and error. However, the pattern of sugar spillage often provides a clue as to what type of insulin will be most effective. Thus, high urine sugars appearing only after meals and disappearing overnight will usually be controlled by a single injection of crystalline insulin. On the other hand, spillage during the day and night is usually not controlled by a single injection and requires either an intermediate type insulin or a mixture of long- and short-acting insulins. The decision in a particular case should lie with the doctor responsible for the care of the patient.

17.*Do you know where to store insulin?*

Insulin should always be kept cold. If it is warmed beyond room temperature the character of the protein changes and it is no longer as effective in lowering the blood sugar.

18. *Filling an insulin syringe properly.*

The withdrawal of insulin from the bottle is best learned by actual demonstration carried out in a doctor's office or in a clinic. In this way bacterial contamination and undesirable mixing of insulin in the bottle when two types are used together can be avoided. The sequence of procedures has been described in Chapter 5 of this book.

19. *Where should insulin be injected?*

If there is no swelling or loss of flesh at injection sites, rotation from arm, to leg, to abdomen, and to buttocks may be freely used. In children and in women, in whom loss of flesh is most apt to occur, it may be desirable to limit the injections to one site or inject the insulin deep into the muscle.

20. *Do you adjust your insulin dosage in accordance with the results of urine tests?*

There is nothing more practical than the urine sugar in evaluating the effectiveness of treatment. The only exception is in those patients who present special problems, particularly those in whom urine tests do not reflect the blood sugar accurately. In general, spillage occurring predominantly during the daytime necessitates more short-acting or more intermediate insulin; that occurring predominantly during the night requires more long-acting or at times more intermediate insulin.

21. *Recognition of insulin shocks.*

It is important to keep in mind that shocking may not always be dramatic. It may, for example, manifest itself only by headaches, malaise, or peculiar sensations on arising. This points to excessive insulin action during the night. It is true, however, that during the day feelings of nervousness, confusion, sweating, or drowsiness are the usual signs. It should be remembered that with longer-acting insulin the nervousness and sweating may be less marked.

22.*Is insulin reaction or shock dangerous?*

Because the brain and the nervous system can use only sugar for energy purposes, anything that lowers the blood sugar below normal interferes with their normal function. This is why drowsiness, loss of consciousness, and convulsions appear in severe insulin shock. Insulin reactions should be viewed as highly undesirable and dangerous. Prolonged lowering of the blood sugar may produce hemorrhage in the brain and may even prove fatal. Other tissues also require a normal blood-sugar level for adequate function. Hence, diet, insulin dosage and the total program of the patient who shocks should be evaluated so that such episodes can be prevented.

23.*Should insulin be stopped if food and fluids cannot be retained?*

The patient who is not taking food or fluids is still obtaining energy from the body stores of carbohydrate, fat, and protein. These reactions require insulin just as if the foodstuffs were being made available through eating. Hence, the patient on insulin who cannot eat should still take insulin. The dosage is usually decreased, unless the infection or other illness interfering with the intake of food is at the same time raising the insulin requirement.

24.*How to recognize acidosis or coma.*

The presence of increased amounts of sugar and the appearance of acetone in the urine or on the breath are the first signs. The former is accompanied by increased urination and increased thirst. As acidosis develops, the patient loses his appetite and vomiting usually appears. The latter occurs in about three-fourths of the cases of acidosis and coma. As the acidosis progresses the patient may develop rapid and deep breathing, and become confused or actually lose consciousness. The face is flushed, the lips are dry, and the eyeballs are soft.

25. *Can acidosis-coma be treated at home?*

In general the hospital is the best place to treat this complication. However, under guidance of the doctor the insulin and intravenous fluids which make up the backbone of acidosis and coma therapy may be administered at home when hospitalization is not possible. This deprives the patient, however, of the margins of safety present in the hospital should an emergency develop.

26. *How may acidosis-coma be prevented?*

Insufficient insulin, infections, emotional upsets, or even insulin shock may precipitate acidosis and coma. Hence, adjustment of insulin dosage to actual need under all of these circumstances is the keystone of prevention. These are times when the advice of the physician or clinic is particularly valuable.

27. *Are operations dangerous?*

The patient can tolerate almost all general and local anesthetics just as well as the nondiabetic. Adjustment of insulin dosage and injection of glucose prior to, during, and after surgery maintains normal energy metabolism. Usually the patient is shifted to short-acting insulin and the blood sugar is used more often as an index during this period of time. With simple surgical procedures, however, the patient may be continued on his usual insulin program.

28. *Is the patient more susceptible to infections?*

In the past it was believed that boils and other surface infections occur more often in diabetes. This may well not be true, except that affected females are more prone to develop infections of the external genitals. The latter arises from irritation by sugar in the urine. Insofar as internal infections are concerned, tuberculosis which used to be common in the patient has decreased greatly. **Urinary-tract infections in diabetes especially in females,** continue to be more frequent than in others and should receive vigorous treatment.

29. *What are shin spots?*

Long-standing diabetes may be associated with the presence of superficial pigmented indentations of various shapes and sizes, generally small, on the lower legs. They are of no practical importance. They are not to be confused with the generally larger spots which represent necrobiosis.

30. *Is coma in the diabetic always due to insulin excess or to keto-acidosis?*

No. These are the most common causes, but coma can develop for other reasons unrelated or related to the diabetes. Thus, it may be incidental, as with brain injury or poisoning, or result from a shortage of oxygen in the tissues (lactic acidosis) or very high levels of sugar or sodium in the blood (hyperosmolar coma).

18 : GLOSSARY FOR PATIENTS

Aceto-acetic acid: ketone bodies produced from fat when insulin or carbohydrate supplies are insufficient as in ketosis or starvation; gives rise to acetone.

Acetone: a breakdown product of fat found in increased amounts in body fluids and in urine when the tissues, unable to obtain sufficient energy from carbohydrate as in untreated diabetes or during starvation, mobilize fat for this purpose.

Acidosis-coma: a major disturbance of the metabolism of foodstuffs in a patient with increased levels of sugar and ketone bodies in the blood and losses of sugar, ketone bodies, water and the chief minerals in urine; acidosis-coma results from an insufficiency of insulin secondary to infection, poor regulation, emotional upsets or even insulin shocking.

Adrenals: cap-shaped endocrine or ductless glands which sit on the upper pole of the kidneys; the innermost part secretes adrenalin which raises the blood sugar by converting glycogen to glucose and stopping insulin secretion. The outer part manufactures steroids which are related to cortisone in structure and in effects; among other actions, these hormones regulate the exchanges of the chief minerals and the water of the body, control the metabolism of foodstuffs, and determine in part certain sex characteristics; excesses of these hormones produce or aggravate diabetes.

Alkali: A solution used to correct the acidosis of acidosis-coma; this is a sodium-containing salt.

Alpha cells: located in the islets of the pancreas; the probable site of glucagon (blood-sugar raising principle) production.

American Diabetes Association: a voluntary health agency composed of physicians, teachers, and research workers in diabetes and lay volunteers. It sponsors professional meetings and the publications, encourages case findings and disseminates information in this field; the association also includes numerous affiliated groups of patients and their families in various areas of the United States; it publishes the journal *Diabetes* for physicians and research workers and the ADA *Forecast,* a bi-monthly journal for diabetics, supplies identification cards for patients, and has available a useful booklet entitled "Facts About Diabetes" (600 Fifth Avenue, New York City 10020).

ADA (American Diabetes Association and American Dietetic Association) diets: these simplify the life of the patient by using tables of food exchanges which in measured amounts contain the same quantity of carbohydrate, fat or protein; available through your doctor or clinic.

ADA *Forecast*: a bi-monthly periodical for patients and their families issued by the American Diabetics Association, 18

East 48th Street, New York City; it is an extremely useful source of valuable information.

Benedict's solution: a preparation of copper sulfate used in tests for glucose and other reducing substances in urine.

Beta cells: site of insulin production in the pancreas.

Carbohydrate: sugars and materials capable of directly giving rise to sugars such as the large molecules of starch, glycogen etc. present in foods; carbohydrates are also formed in the body from protein and from the glycerol part of fat; the individual molecules consist of carbon hydrogen and water, and hence the term carbohydrate; simple sugars of importance in human metabolism include glucose, fructose, ribose, and galactose; table sugar is a "double sugar" or disaccharide and is made up of glucose and fructose linked together; "milk sugar" or lactose consists of glucose and galactose, and maltose used in malted milk shakes consists of 2 molecules of glucose; the metabolism of 1 gram of carbohydrate to carbon dioxide and water releases 4 calories of energy.

Carbon dioxide of serum (or, less accurately, serum carbondioxide combining power): an important index employed in the diagnosis and treatment of diabetic acidosis and coma.

Clinistix®: pieces of cardboard the size of paper matchsticks impregnated with glucose oxidase, an enzyme which acts only upon glucose, and used for the qualitative identification of glucose; not suitable for measuring the actual amounts present.

Clinitest®: tablets for testing the urine for sugar; these contain a copper salt and alkali which react with urine to produce heat and a color change if glucose or other reducing substances are present.

Coma or loss of consciousness occurring in a patient: may be diabetic acidosis-coma, it can be a severe insulin shock, or it may be totally unrelated to the diabetes, resulting for example from a hemorrhage or other injury to the brain or an excessive dose of sleeping medicine. Other types of coma may also occur, including lactic acidosis due to general or local shortage of oxygen and the hyperosmolar disorders as a result of very high blood glucose or serum sodium levels.

Crystalline insulin: like regular insulin in its blood-sugar controlling effects but a more pure form.

Diabetes insipidus: literally "a flow of non-sweet urine" and therefore not diabetes in the ordinary sense. Diabetes insipidus is a disorder of the water-regulating mechanism of the body and does not affect the metabolism of sugar and other foodstuffs.

Diabetes mellitus: a disturbance in the metabolism of foodstuffs (carbohydrate, fat, and protein) resulting from a relative or absolute shortage of insulin or insulin effects.

Endocrine glands: collections of specialized cells which manufacture hormones that are poured directly into the body fluids and into the blood stream without passing through a system of tubes. Examples: pituitary, thyroid, parathyroid, adrenals, ovaries, testes, and the islet cells of the pancreas; all but the parathyroid glands are known to be capable of influencing the metabolism of foodstuffs.

Enzymes: proteins which effect the breakdown or conversions of foodstuffs in the body; thus the breakdown of glucose to carbon dioxide, water and energy and the conversion of amino acids to glucose is effected by enzymes.

Fasting blood-sugar levels: obtained before breakfast after an all-night fast; if increased above normal, they usually indicate a disturbance of glucose metabolism which may be diabetes.

Fat atrophy: disappearance of fat at sites of insulin injections occurring in certain children and some adult diabetics.

Fats: one of the three major foodstuffs; consist of molecules of carbon, hydrogen and water (occasionally other elements are present as well); about 9 calories of energy are released when 1 gram of fat is broken down to carbon dioxide and water.

Foodstuffs: refer to the three major constituents of food, i.e. the carbohydrates, fats, and proteins.

"Free" diets: also called normal or liberalized diets and used in the treatment of certain patients; under the direction of the doctor some patients may eat practically the same foods that are served to the rest of the family but the amounts taken are regulated, consciously or unconsciously. However, prudent patients first weigh and measure their food and then use ADA diets based on meat, fat, and other exchanges.

Globin insulin: an intermediate type of insulin made with globin, a protein, to retard its action; resembles certain mixtures of protamine zinc and crystalline insulin and is like NPH insulin in intensity and duration of effects.

Glucagon: a protein hormone (produced by the pancreas and cells of the intestinal tract) which raises blood-sugar levels, chiefly by converting liver glycogen to blood sugar.

Glucose solutions: consist of water and various amounts of glucose (5, 10, 50 per cent, etc.) and are used to replace the losses of water which occur in acidosis and coma; glucose solutions may also be injected as an emergency replacement for food in treating insulin shock, or given by mouth or by vein in glucose tolerance tests in diagnosing diabetes.

Glucose tolerance tests: tests during which the effect of a certain amount of glucose upon the blood sugar is determined; the test load of sugar may be given by mouth (oral test) or by vein (intravenous test); used in the diagnosis of diabetes and other disturbances of body metabolism.

Glycogen: a huge molecule of glucose units linked together; the storage form of glucose in the liver, muscles, and other tissues.

Hemoglobin A (glycosylated or $HgbA_{1c}$): hemoglobin present in red cells provides a record of long-term adequate or inadequate control of blood sugar; normally $HgbA_{1c}$ is present in 3 to 6% of the hemoglobin molecules but with inadequate control and high blood sugars this percentage can double.

Insulin: the protein hormone produced by the beta cells of the pancreas which regulates the use of foodstuffs in the body; the ability to lower levels of blood sugar is the best known of these effects.

Ketone bodies: beta-hydroxy butyric acid, aceto-acetic (or diacetic) acid, and a breakdown product of the latter, acetone; ketone bodies are formed from fat in the poorly regulated patient at an excessive rate and therefore accumulate in the blood and appear in the urine; may be the prelude to diabetic acidosis or coma, but also occur with insulin shocks and with inadequate intake of sugars and starches.

Ketosis: an accumulation of ketone bodies in the body fluids of poorly regulated patients as well as in other conditions such as starvation (and insulin shocks); ketosis may progress to acidosis or coma.

Lente insulin: an intermediate insulin; semi-Lente and ultra-Lente have faster and slower actions, respectively.

Mellituria (also spelled melituria): literally, "honey or sweet substance in the urine"; usually glucose but may be one of the other sugars.

NPH insulin: a protamine type of insulin made without an excess of protamine and possessing a peak and duration of action between that of crystalline insulin and PZI; an intermediate-type insulin which may be used in combination with crystalline insulin to obtain a more intense action.

Potassium: the chief mineral inside of cells; losses of potassium as in acidosis-coma interfere with the function and structure of cells; it is given during the treatment of acidosis-coma.

Pre-diabetic syndrome: interval from birth to the first abnormal elevations of blood glucose indicative of diabetes; the tendency for big babies to be born of mothers who are going to develop diabetes later and which can also manifest itself in other ways, such as the inability to carry a pregnancy to the point of the birth of a live baby; the interval prior to diabetes.

Protamine zinc insulin (also called PZI): insulin combined with another protein (protamine) and with zinc to slow the rate of absorption and thereby provide a slower, less intense and more prolonged effect; also called long-acting insulin; may be used in combination with crystalline or regular insulin, but ratio of the two must be two or more parts of crystalline to one part of PZI before crystalline insulin can exert its effects. For this and other reasons PZI insulin is now used only infrequently.

Proteins: carbon, hydrogen, oxygen and nitrogen present in

units known as amino acids (glycine is the simplest: $NH_2\text{-}CH_2COOH$) linked together to form peptides and ultimately proteins via the peptide linkage (-CONH-); certain amino acids must be derived from foods because they cannot be manufactured in the body and are therefore called "essential"; the remainder can be made from sugar and other products of metabolism and are called "non-essential"; both the "essential" and "non-essential" amino acids are necessary, however, for growth and maintenance of the proteins of tissues; when used for energy purposes 1 gram of protein yields 4 calories; the ordinary American diet provides about 1 gram per 2.2 pounds of body weight, though under most circumstances of health less than this is adequate.

PZI insulin: see Protamine Zinc insulin.

Regular insulin: noncrystalline insulin obtained from the pancreas of animals and possessing a rapid onset and short, 6-to-8-hour, duration of action.

Renal diabetes (also called renal glycosuria or true renal glucosuria): a "leakage" of sugar by the kidneys despite the fact that blood-sugar levels are normal; should not be called diabetes since there is no disturbance of the metabolism of sugar or other foodstuffs.

Saccharin: this artificial sweetener as well as the cyclamates are restricted for general use but are available to diabetics; the restrictions stem from the law that any agent that causes cancer in animals can not be in general use.

Sodium: the chief mineral in the body fluids which surround the cells; excessive losses of sodium as in acidosis and coma result in a loss of circulatory efficiency with decreased pumping of blood by the heart, drop in blood pressure, etc.

Swelling at site of insulin injections: a reaction to insulin occurring in some children and certain adults with diabetes.

Tes-Tape®: a roll of paper which contains glucose oxidase; solutions of glucose change the yellow color to various shades of green or blue, depending on the amounts present.

Thyroid: an endocrine gland in the neck which secretes thyroxin (T_4) and triiodothyronine (T_3); overactivity of this gland makes diabetes worse.

Tolerance tests: measurements of the ability of the body to dispose of or "tolerate" test amounts of certain substances such as glucose.

Vascular disease: changes in the blood vessels of the body as in the feet, the eyes, the kidney, etc.

APPENDIX

1. Detailed instructions for urine sugar tests

A. CLINITEST®

The manufacturer of Clinitest®, Ames Company, Inc. of Elkhart, Indiana, provides the following information for the use of these tablets of copper sulfate, caustic soda, sodium carbonate and citric acid in the determination of urine sugar without heating or boiling:

Collect urine in clean receptacle. With dropper in upright position, place 5 drops urine in test tube. Rinse dropper and place 10 drops of water in the test tube. Drop 1 tablet into test tube. *Watch while reaction takes place.* (See interpretation of test.) Do not shake test tube during reaction nor for 15 seconds after boiling inside test tube has stopped. After 15-second waiting period, shake test tube gently and compare with color scale.

189

Interpretation of Clinitest results: *Negative:* no sugar (glucose)—the fluid will be blue at the end of a waiting period of 15 seconds. All shades of blue are negative. The whitish sediment that may form has no bearing on the test. *Positive:* sugar present—the fluid will change color. The more sugar, the greater the change and the more rapidly it occurs.

An amount of sugar over 2% causes rapid color changes to green, tan, orange and finally to a dark shade of greenish brown, which should not be confused with any color on the chart. Sometimes, when the amount of sugar is very large this final change takes place before the 15-second wait is over—hence the necessity of watching the reaction. Should the fluid even fleetingly pass through orange to dark greenish-brown, record as over 2% without comparing with the color scale. The color scale supplied indicates the following:

dark blue	(no sugar)	−0%	Insignificant losses of sugar
dark green	(trace)	−¼%	
olive green	(1+)	−½%	
green brown	(2+)	−¾%	Moderate losses of sugar
tan brown	(3+)	−1%	
red orange	(4+)	−2% or more	Marked losses of sugar

B. TES-TAPE ®

Remove approximately one and one-half inches of Tes-Tape. Then dip in specimen; remove and wait one minute, compare darkest area with chart supplied on container by the manufacturer, Eli Lilly and company:

yellow	(no sugar)	−0%	
light green	(1+)	−1/10%	Interpretation as above but
dark green	(2+)	−¼%	note that it is not always
green blue	(3+)	−½%	possible to measure values
dark blue	(4+)	−2% or more	between ½ and 2%. Waiting an extra minute helps.

C. KETO-DIASTIX®

A Keto-Diastix® strip dipped into urine for 2 seconds yields a glucose value of 1/10, 1/4, 1/2, 1, or 2% or more in 30 seconds and an acetone reading (small, moderate, or large) in just 15 seconds. The sugar test material is glucose oxidase and peroxidase. The acetone test is based on the usual nitroprusside reaction. A purple color develops when acetone or acetoacetic acid is present but it does not detect the other ketone body, beta hydroxybutyric acid. With both tests exact timing is essential.

D. CHEMSTRIP®

Brodynamics/BMC provides a striptest for glucose, ketones and other urine constitutents. The glucose test employs oxidase and peroxidase and is semi-quantitative. The ketone test measures only acetone and acetoacetic acid.

E. CLINISTIX®

Clinistix® paper, supplied by Ames Company Inc. of Elkhart, Indiana, contains glucose oxidase and is useful for determining whether a particular reducing substance in urine is really glucose, but at present it cannot be used to determine the concentration of sugar:

1. Dip test end of Clinistix in urine and remove (or moisten with a drop of urine).
2. Positive: Moistened end turns blue. Negative: No blue color develops. (Check both sides of strip.)

    When sugar is present blue color normally appears in less than a minute, but occasionally may be delayed a minute or so, depending on nature of urine.

2. The intensity and duration of action of the various insulins

A. "REGULAR" OR "CRYSTALLINE" (CLEAR SOLUTION)

The insulin used by Banting and Best in their studies in animals and in humans was by today's standards an extremely crude and weak extract of the pancreas. Through the years steady progress has been made in obtaining a successively more pure preparation of insulin. The early forms of insulin were called "regular" and lowered the blood sugar, keeping it low for 6 to 8 hours. By the 1930's insulin was pure enough to be crystallized out of solution and hence the introduction of the term "crytalline." Insofar as control of diabetes is concerned, the regular and crystalline insulins have always been interchangeable in terms or rapid onset and short duration of action. Because of these properties, and in view of the introduction of the newer insulins, these two are now designated as short-acting. The crystalline type is less apt to produce allergic reactions.

Short-acting insulins usually necessitate two or more injections each day to control the blood and urine sugar throughout the entire twenty-four hours. Though patients with infections or other acute illnesses, those in acidosis or coma, and many undergoing surgery, required and still require rapid-acting insulin several times each day, routine control could usually be managed with only two injections of either of these two insulins. These were given before breakfast and before supper. Since the first injection of the day had to provide coverage for two meals, the usual dosage was about twice that taken just prior to the evening meal.

B. THE FIRST OF THE LONGER-ACTING INSULINS: PROTAMINE ZINC OR "PZI" (CLOUDY SOLUTION)

In 1936 Hagedorn, a Scandinavian scientist, announced that the addition of zinc and a protein derived from fish to short-acting insulin decreased the intensity of the blood-sugar lowering effect but prolonged the action to twenty-four hours or longer. This was related to the slower absorption of the PZI complex compared to the short-acting forms. It soon became apparent that this long-acting insulin could provide effective control when given alone to certain patients requiring up to 60 units or so each day. In the remainder the after-meal rise in blood and urine sugar could not be prevented without precipitating an insulin shock during the night. It was logical to test, therefore, the effects of mixtures of the short- and long-acting insulins.

C. THE USE OF PZI IN COMBINATION WITH REGULAR OR CRYSTALLINE INSULIN

It was soon established that if PZI and crystalline or regular insulin were mixed together in one bottle in equal proportions, the intensity and the duration of PZI was not detectably altered. However, mixtures of two parts or more of the short-acting insulin to one part of PZI properly adjusted for the individual patient did provide better coverage of the after-meal rise and spill of sugar without producing a nighttime insulin shock. The answer to this phenomenon lay in the fact that PZI contains extra or unused protamine which can and does unite with the added crystalline insulin and thereby produces more PZI. Once all of this excess protamine is used up, one can expect and does see the after-meal effect of the short-acting insulin. It is obvious, of course, that if the two types of insulin are injected separately into two different areas rather than premixed in the bottle the action of each will be manifest. This has been the custom in certain clinics, though it does require two different injections. Some patients have "layered" the two insulins in a single syringe and, after introducing the needle under the skin, have injected them into two nearby, though different, sites. Others mix the insulins in the syringe and inject them into one area.

Protamine insulin used in conjunction with a short-acting insulin in either one of the three schemes described above has been a great boon in the regulation of diabetes. With a single injection of these two insulins before breakfast, full 24-hour control of diabetes can be obtained. This has been the chief method of insulin therapy during the years preceding the introduction of globin, NPH, and the lente insulins. It should be pointed out, however, that in some clinics it has been the practice to give the PZI at a later time in the day, usually before supper. This is also a satisfactory schedule, since the general experience indicates that PZI exerts its steady low-intensity effect quite evenly during the twenty-four hours no matter when it is given. It is, however, less convenient.

D. THE REASON FOR GLOBIN (CLEAR) AND NPH (CLOUDY) INSULINS; USE OF NPH AND SHORT-ACTING FORMS

By 1940 and 1950 respectively, two new insulin preparations were available as substitutes for the most frequently used regular or crystalline: PZI mixture, the 2:1. The first of these was called globin insulin. Its intensity and duration of action fell between those of the rapid-acting and the long-acting insulins. This has proved quite satisfactory for the control of certain patients. This same general statement applies to the NPH insulin which is a protamine zinc insulin made without excess protamine. It is obvious, however, since 2:1 mixtures did not meet the needs of all patients, that substitutes for 2:1 mixtures would not do so either. Hence mixtures of NPH and short-acting insulin were introduced to take care of patients needing 3:1, 4:1 mixtures, etc.

E. THE NEWEST OF THE INSULINS: THE LENTE SERIES (CLOUDY SOLUTIONS)

In an attempt to provide an insulin which would meet the needs of more and more patients, the solution in which insulin is ordinarily dissolved was changed and the lente (*lente*—slow) series was evolved. This in general resembles the 2:1 short-acting and PZI mixture, the globin, and the NPH preparations, but it can be modified to give a more rapid and more intense action (semi-lente insulin) or a slower and more prolonged effect (ultra-lente).

3. The role of the pituitary, thyroid, and other glands in diabetes

A. THE PITUITARY GLAND

Patients with tumors of the pink-staining cells, the eosinophils, of the pituitary gland which is located at the base of the brain and has been called the master gland, may develop diabetes. The actual incidence of diabetes in such patients ranges from 20 to 40 per cent in the experience of the various clinics and hospitals. These pituitary tumors produce growth hormone which simultaneously accelerates the output of insulin by the pancreas and interferes with the action of insulin in the tissues. It would appear that patients whose reserves of ability to manufacture insulin are low are the ones who develop diabetes. However, this physiologically informative experiment on the part of nature has no practical significance in the life of more than 99 per cent of patients. They do not have eosinophil tumors of the pituitary nor is there any evidence that in ordinary diabetes the eosinophils are working overtime in producing this hormone. The physician can quickly decide about the possibility of such a tumor just by looking at the patient, because the hormone produces characteristic changes in the bones and soft tissues which have been called acromegaly. His judgment can then be supported by measurements of the levels of growth hormone in serum. If the physician happens to see such a patient, and they are so rare that it is usual for a doctor not to see even one during an entire lifetime of practice, a program of evaluation and of treatment can be worked out which can not only cancel some of the soft tissue and bone changes but also lessen the severity of the diabetes.

However, temporary excesses of growth hormone often develop many times during the day and night when insulin-treated diabetes is incompletely controlled. These do not produce any signs of acromegaly but could contribute to eye and kidney problems.

B. THE THYROID

Real overactivity of the thyroid gland will aggravate diabetes which was present previously or was about to develop anyway. This relationship has been recognized for years by physicians and is among the possibilities considered whenever diabetes becomes worse and the search for all of the usual causes of such aggravation has been fruitless.

This sequence can be best illustrated perhaps by citing the case history of a diabetic patient who developed over-activity of the thyroid gland. This lady, L.M., was thirty-four years old when she noted the onset of a 15-pound weight loss, increased appetite, increased thirst and increased voiding. The urine contained sugar and the fasting blood sugar was increased. She responded to treatment consisting of a diabetic diet and insulin. She required up to 20 units of insulin each day. Fourteen months later she noted that, despite the fact she was following the diet closely, the urine sugar and the insulin requirement were both rising until she was taking as much as 100 units each day. When she came to the diabetic clinic the physician checked her for evidences of infection and inquired about her personal affairs but found nothing wrong. On examination the thyroid gland proved to be enlarged and the patient showed several signs which suggested that this gland was overactive. Appropriate laboratory tests during a period in the hospital proved this to be true. She received treatment which returned the gland to normal activity and simultaneously her insulin requirement fell back to its previous low level.

There are a number of reasons why thyroid overactivity raises the insulin requirement and makes it more difficult to regulate blood and urine sugars. First, such patients become hungry and eat a great deal more. This introduces a greater load of carbohydrate and other foodstuffs which must be covered by increased dosages of insulin. Then, the excesses of thyroid hormone alter the orderly absorption of food stuffs from the gastrointestinal tract. Also, the excretion of sugar by the kidneys is changed in this condition. These last two factors serve to complicate the use of blood and urine sugar levels in the regulation of diabetes. Moreover, in thyroid overactivity the emergency stores of glucose in the liver in the form of glycogen are often greatly decreased. This makes diabetic control difficult because between meals the body cannot draw on its usual stores of glucose to cover the insulin which has been injected. Also, when the liver is low in glycogen it tends to make more ketone bodies than usual. There are a number of other ways in which thyroid overactivity influences the metabolism of foodstuffs such as the losses of body protein, the altered disposal of sugar in tissues, and the increased destruction of injected insulin which need not be discussed in detail. The final net effect of all these factors in an increase in the severity of the diabetes.

If thyroid overactivity has increased the severity of the diabetes, return of the thyroid gland to normal will be followed by a decrease in insulin requirement and once again make regulation easier. Today there are many effective ways of treating thyroid overactivity. The physician is guided by the type of thyroid overactivity, the age of the patient, the presence of complications such as heart disease and similar factors, in deciding which therapy is best suited for a particular patient.

C. THE ADRENAL

Tumors of the innermost part of the adrenal, *i.e.*, the medulla, usually raise the blood pressure and may by themselves produce elevations of the blood sugar and a spillage of sugar in the urine in some patients. These are called pheochromocytomas. Such tumors put out large amounts of adrenalin and closely related secretions which act to convert liver and other tissue glycogen to glucose, interfere with the use of glucose by the tissues, stop the secretion of insulin by the islet cells of the pancreas, and thereby affect carbohydrate metabolism. In diabetes they make control difficult. Fortunately this is quite a rare problem in the population in general and is of no importance to those with diabetes as a whole. If high blood pressure appears in a patient and the diabetes becomes worse, the physician can look for the possible presence of such a tumor by several procedures, some of them quite simple.

Overactivity or tumors of the outer part of the adrenal gland, the cortex, may also produce or increase the severity of a diabetes. Larger-than-normal amounts of steroids of the cortisol type are manufactured and released into the blood stream. Some of these steroids increase the rate of new formation of glucose and interfere with the action of insulin in tissues. Again, these are very rare occurrences in individuals with or without diabetes, and if the question is raised it can only be resolved by detailed studies.

D. GLUCAGON

The alpha cells of the pancreas and other tissues secrete glucagon, a hormone which raises blood sugar levels by converting liver glycogen to glucose. Tumors which produce glucagon, called glucagonomas, result in diabetes. They are extremely rare. When removed, the diabetes usually disappears.

4. Roster of lay diabetes societies

AMERICAN DIABETES ASSOCIATION, INC.
600 Fifth Avenue
New York, New York 10020
212 541-4310

ALABAMA
AMERICAN DIABETES
ASSOCIATION
ALABAMA AFFILIATE
904 Bob Wallace Avenue, S.E.
Huntsville, Alabama 35801

ALASKA
8130 Buckleberry
Anchorage, Alaska 99502

ARIZONA
ARIZONA DIABETES
ASSOCIATION
555 West Catalina Drive
Phoenix, Arizona 85013

4901 E. Fifth Street
Tuscon, Arizona 85716

ARKANSAS
AMERICAN DIABETES
ASSOCIATION
ARKANSAS AFFILIATE
5422 West Markham
Little Rock, Arkansas 72205

CALIFORNIA
AMERICAN DIABETES
ASSOCIATION
NORTHERN CALIFORNIA
AFFILIATE
255 Hugo Street
San Francisco, California 94122

AMERICAN DIABETES
ASSOCIATION
NORTHERN CALIFORNIA
AFFILIATE

4383 Piedmont Avenue
Oakland, California 94611

1st Methodist Church
9 Ross Valley Drive
San Rafael, California 94901

Central Methodist Church
5265 H Street
Sacramento, California 95819

AMERICAN DIABETES
ASSOCIATION
SOUTHERN CALIFORNIA
AFFILIATE
1127 Crenshaw Boulevard
Los Angeles, California 90019

3420 Kenyon Street
San Diego, California 92110

1215 East Chapman Avenue
Orange, California 92666

COLORADO
AMERICAN DIABETES
ASSOCIATION
COLORADO AFFILIATE
1045 Acoma Street
Denver, Colorado 80204

CONNECTICUT
AMERICAN DIABETES
ASSOCIATION
CONNECTICUT AFFILIATE
17 Oakwood Avenue
West Hartford, Connecticut 06119

DELAWARE
AMERICAN DIABETES
ASSOCIATION
DELAWARE AFFILIATE
2300 Pennsylvania Avenue
Wilmington, Delaware 19806

DISTRICT OF COLUMBIA
AMERICAN DIABETES
ASSOCIATION
WASHINGTON, D.C. AREA
AFFILIATE

7961 Eastern Avenue
Silver Spring, Maryland 20910

FLORIDA
AMERICAN DIABETES
ASSOCIATION
FLORIDA AFFILIATE
930 Cesery Boulevard
Jacksonville Florida 32211

GEORGIA
AMERICAN DIABETES
ASSOCIATION
GEORGIA AFFILIATE
1447 Peachtree Street N.E.
Atlanta, Georgia 30309

HAWAII
AMERICAN DIABETES
ASSOCIATION
HAWAII AFFILIATE
347 N. Kuahini Street
Honolulu, Hawaii 96817

IDAHO
AMERICAN DIABETES
ASSOCIATION
IDAHO AFFILIATE
P.O. Box 71123
Boise, Idaho 83707

ILLINOIS
AMERICAN DIABETES
ASSOCIATION
NORTHERN ILLINOIS
AFFILIATE
620 North Michigan Avenue
Chicago, Illinois 60611

AMERICAN DIABETES
ASSOCIATION
DOWNSTATE ILLINOIS
AFFILIATE
104 North Water
Decatur, Illinois 62523

INDIANA
AMERICAN DIABETES
ASSOCIATION
INDIANA AFFILIATE

222 S. Downey Avenue
Indianapolis, Indiana 46219

1433 North Meridian Street
Indianapolis, Indiana 46202

IOWA
AMERICAN DIABETES
ASSOCIATION
IOWA AFFILIATE
305 Second Avenue, S.E.
Cedar Rapids, Iowa 52401

KANSAS
AMERICAN DIABETES
ASSOCIATION
KANSAS AFFILIATE
2312 East Central
Wichita, Kansas 67214

KENTUCKY
AMERICAN DIABETES
ASSOCIATION
KENTUCKY AFFILIATE
2358 Pierson Drive
Lexington, Kentucky 40505

LOUISIANA
AMERICAN DIABETES
ASSOCIATION
LOUISIANA AFFILIATE
619 Building
619 Jefferson Highway
Baton Rouge, Louisiana 70816

MAINE
See Massachusetts

MARYLAND
AMERICAN DIABETES
ASSOCIATION
MARYLAND AFFILIATE
3701 Old Court Road
Old Court Executive Park,
Baltimore, Maryland 21208

MASSACHUSETTS
AMERICAN DIABETES
ASSOCIATION
NEW ENGLAND AFFILIATE

377 Elliot Street
Newton Upper Falls, Massachusetts 02164

MICHIGAN
AMERICAN DIABETES
ASSOCIATION
MICHIGAN AFFILIATE
6131 West Outer Drive
Detroit, Michigan 48235

MINNESOTA
AMERICAN DIABETES
ASSOCIATION
MINNESOTA AFFILIATE
7601 Bush Lake Road
Minneapolis, Minnesota 55435

6490 Excelsior Boulevard
W-414 Meadowbrook Building
St. Louis Park, Minnesota 55426

MISSISSIPPI
AMERICAN DIABETES
ASSOCIATION
MISSISSIPPI AFFILIATE
P.O. Box 16968
Jackson, Mississippi 39206

MISSOURI
AMERICAN DIABETES
ASSOCIATION
HEART OF AMERICA
AFFILIATE
616 East 63rd Street
Kansas City, Missouri 64110

AMERICAN DIABETES
ASSOCIATION
MISSOURI REGIONAL
AFFILIATE
Box 11
Columbia, Missouri 65201

AMERICAN DIABETES
ASSOCIATION
GREATER ST. LOUIS
AFFILIATE
3839 Lindell Boulevard
St. Louis, Missouri 63108

MONTANA
  AMERICAN DIABETES
  ASSOCIATION
  MONTANA AFFILIATE
  Box 2411
  Great Falls, Montana 59403

NEBRASKA
  AMERICAN DIABETES
  ASSOCIATION
  NEBRASKA AFFILIATE
  819 Dorcas Street
  Omaha, Nebraska 68108

NEVADA
  AMERICAN DIABETES
  ASSOCIATION
  NEVADA AFFILIATE
  3333 West Washington Avenue
  Las Vegas, Nevada 89107

NEW HAMPSHIRE
  AMERICAN DIABETES
  ASSOCIATION
  NEW HAMPSHIRE AFFILIATE
  P.O. Box 1312
  Concord, New Hampshire 03301

NEW JERSEY
  AMERICAN DIABETES
  ASSOCIATION
  NEW JERSEY AFFILIATE
  American Red Cross Building
  345 Union Street
  Hackensack, New Jersey 07601

NEW MEXICO
  AMERICAN DIABETES
  ASSOCIATION
  NEW MEXICO AFFILIATE
  6101 Marble, N.E.,
  Albuquerque, New Mexico 87110

NEW YORK
  AMERICAN DIABETES
  ASSOCIATION
  UPPER HUDSON AREA
  CHAPTER
  35 Hackett Avenue
  Albany, New York 12205

AMERICAN DIABETES
ASSOCIATION
WESTERN NEW YORK
AFFILIATE
Statler Hilton
107 Delaware Avenue,
Buffalo, New York 14202

NEW YORK DIABETES
ASSOCIATION
104 East 40th Street
New York, New York 10016

ROCHESTER REGIONAL
DIABETES ASSOCIATION
1351 Mount Hope Avenue
Rochester, New York 14620

AMERICAN DIABETES
ASSOCIATION
UPSTATE NEW YORK
CHAPTER
710 Wilson Building
306 South Salina Street
Syracuse, New York 13202

AMERICAN DIABETES
ASSOCIATION
CENTRAL NEW YORK
CHAPTER
1404 Genesee Street
Utica, New York 13502

NORTH CAROLINA
  AMERICAN DIABETES
  ASSOCIATION
  NORTH CAROLINA AFFILIATE
  408 North Tryon Street
  Charlotte, North Carolina 28202

NORTH DAKOTA
  AMERICAN DIABETES
  ASSOCIATION
  NORTH DAKOTA AFFILIATE
  P.O. Box 234
  Grand Forks, North Dakota 58201

OHIO
  AMERICAN DIABETES
  ASSOCIATION

AKRON AREA AFFILIATE
225 West Exchange Street
Akron, Ohio 44302

AMERICAN DIABETES
ASSOCIATION
CINCINNATI AFFILIATE
2400 Reading Road
Cincinnati, Ohio 45202

AMERICAN DIABETES
ASSOCIATION
DAYTON AREA AFFILIATE
184 Salem Avenue
Dayton, Ohio 45406

AMERICAN DIABETES
ASSOCIATION
MAHONING VALLEY
CHAPTER
420 Oak Hill Avenue
Youngstown, Ohio 44502

AMERICAN DIABETES
ASSOCIATION
SOUTHEASTERN OHIO
CHAPTER
Box 2354
Zanesville, Ohio 43701

OKLAHOMA
AMERICAN DIABETES
ASSOCIATION
EASTERN OKLAHOMA
CHAPTER,
6565 South Yale Avenue,
Tulsa, Oklahoma 74136

AMERICAN DIABETES
ASSOCIATION
WESTERN OKLAHOMA
CHAPTER
2801 N.W. Expressway,
Oklahoma City, Oklahoma 73112

OREGON
AMERICAN DIABETES
ASSOCIATION
OREGON AFFILIATE
3607 S.W. Corbett
Portland, Oregon 97201

PENNSYLVANIA
AMERICAN DIABETES
ASSOCIATION
GREATER PHILADELPHIA
AFFILIATE
919 Walnut Street,
Philadelphia, Pennsylvania 19107

AMERICAN DIABETES
ASSOCIATION
WESTERN PENNSYLVANIA
AFFILIATE
4401 5th Avenue
Pittsburgh, Pennsylvania 15213

AMERICAN DIABETES
ASSOCIATION
PENNSYLVANIA AFFILIATE
739 Hamilton Mall,
Allentown, Pennsylvania 18101

RHODE ISLAND
See Massachusetts

SOUTH CAROLINA
AMERICAN DIABETES
ASSOCIATION
SOUTH CAROLINA
AFFILIATE
P.O. Box 6562
745 No. Pleasantburg Drive
Greenville, South Carolina 29606

SOUTH DAKOTA
AMERICAN DIABETES
ASSOCIATION
SOUTH DAKOTA
AFFILIATE
P.O. Box 1842
Aberdeen, South Dakota 57401

TENNESSEE
AMERICAN DIABETES
ASSOCIATION
GREATER CHATTANOOGA
CHAPTER
871 McCallie Avenue
Chattanooga, Tennessee 37403

AMERICAN DIABETES
ASSOCIATION

KNOX AREA UNIT
815 Broadway, N.E.
Knoxville, Tennessee 37917

AMERICAN DIABETES
ASSOCIATION
MEMPHIS MID-SOUTH
CHAPTER
969 Madison Avenue,
Memphis, Tennessee 38104

AMERICAN DIABETES
ASSOCIATION
MIDDLE TENNESSEE
CHAPTER
c/o Baptist Hospital
Room 120, West Building
2000 Church Street
Nashville, Tennessee 37236

TEXAS
AMERICAN DIABETES
ASSOCIATION
NORTH TEXAS AFFILIATE
P.O. Box 35785
5415 Maple, Dallas, Texas 75235

AMERICA DIABETES
ASSOCIATION
SOUTH TEXAS AFFILIATE
1536 East Anderson Lane
Austin, Texas 78752

4101 Medical Parkway
Austin, Texas 77098

2990 Richmond,
Houston, Texas 77098

UTAH
AMERICAN DIABETES
ASSOCIATION
UTAH AFFILIATE
Graystone Plaza, #4

1174 East 2700 South
Salt Lake City, Utah 84106

VERMONT
AMERICAN DIABETES
ASSOCIATION
VERMONT AFFILIATE
106 Colchester Avenue
Burlington, Vermont 05401

VIRGINIA
AMERICAN DIABETES
ASSOCIATION
VIRGINIA AFFILIATE
210 Laskin Road,
Virginia Beach, Virginia 23451

WASHINGTON
AMERICAN DIABETES
ASSOCIATION
WASHINGTON AFFILIATE
1218 Terry Avenue,
Seattle, Washington 98101

WEST VIRGINIA
AMERICAN DIABETES
ASSOCIATION
WEST VIRGINIA AFFILIATE
1036 Quarrier Street,
Charleston, West Virginia 25301

WISCONSIN
AMERICAN DIABETES
ASSOCIATION
WISCONSIN AFFILIATE
P.O. Box 17805
5215 North Ironwood Road
Milwaukee, Wisconsin 53217

WYOMING
AMERICAN DIABETES
ASSOCIATION
CHEYENNE UNIT
DePaul Hospital
2600 East 18th Street
Cheyenne, Wyoming 82001

INDEX

Acetest®, 40–41
Aceto-acetic acid, 180
Acetone. *See* Ketone bodies
Acetone, testing for, 40–41
Acetone Test Denco®, 41
Acidosis. *See* Acidosis-coma
Acidosis-coma: antecedent events, 108; as a cause of unconsciousness,
   113; as an advanced stage of diabetes, 27–28; as differentiated from
   insulin shock, 114–16; causes of, 106–7; chemical disturbance in,
   110; concern for, 110; in adults, 106; in children, 105; preventing,
   107–8; recovering from, 111; risks of, 105–6; signs of, 106–9, 114;
   treating, 111–12. *See also* Diabetes, living with
Acromegaly, R #197
ADA diets, 59–64
Adrenal gland: as aggravator of diabetes, 98; in reducing severity of
   diabetes, 103
Adrenalin, in treating insulin shock, 117–18
Alcoholic beverages, 147
Atrophy. *See* Insulin injections

Between-meal feedings. *See* Diets, diabetic
Birth control pills and diabetic control, 94
Blood sugar level: in acidosis-coma, 112; in controlling diabetes, 36; in
   digestion, 18–19; in loss of consciousness, 114–15; in preventing
   cataracts, 125; in various stages of diabetes, 24 ff. *See also* Insulin,
   how it functions; Glucose testing; Urine analysis
Blood vessel problems in diabetes, 130–32. *See also* Diabetes, living
   with

Caloric requirements in diabetic diet, 48–50
Carbohydrate intake in diabetic diets, 49–52
Carbutamide®, 86
Chemical diabetes, 26
Clinistix®, 38–40
Clinitest®, 38–40, 146, 182
Consciousness, loss of: causes, 113, 183; differentiation of causes, 116–
   17, types, 183

Diabetes: aggravating, 92–99; attitudes toward, 17–18, 20–22, 122–23;
   causes, 18, 41; chemical, 26, curing, 100–4; diagnosis of, 33;
   early detection in preventing acidosis-coma, 107; female susceptibility
   to, 17; glossary of terms for, 180 ff.; hereditary influences, 20; how
   it begins, 20; metabolic changes in, 15; onset in adults, 28–29; onset
   in children, 28–29, 151; precautions, 119; questions and answers re-
   garding, 169–79; reducing severity of, 101–3; special problems in,
   122–33; stages of, 24 ff.; symptoms of well-controlled, 45; symptoms
   of uncontrolled, 41–45; testing for, 20, 33–35
Diabetes, controlling: during pregnancy, 157–58; effect of irregular
   diet, 95–97; effect of irregular insulin injections, 96–97; role of doctor, 22–23, 122; role of family, 22–23, 122; use of blood sugar levels,
   36–37; use of urine sugar levels, 36–37. *See also* Diets, diabetic; Infections in diabetes; Insulin injections; Insulin substitutes
Diabetes, living with: attitudes, 161–64; expectations, 164–68
Diabetes, social aspects of, 141 ff.; alcoholic beverages, 147; dating,
   145–46; responsibility of hostess, 141–44; responsibility of housewife, 144; traveling, 146–47
Diabetes, temporary stress-induced, as a stage of diabetes, 25
Diabetes, treating. *See* Diets, diabetic; Insulin; Insulin substitutes
Diabetes in children, 148 ff.; age of onset, 28–29, 151; causes of, 149;
   familial cases, 150; first signs, 152–53; results of proper treatment,
   155; susceptibility, 149; treating, 48, 154–55
Diabetes insipidus, definition, 15
Diabetes mellitus, definition, 15
Diabetes pre-mellitus. *See* Pre-diabetes